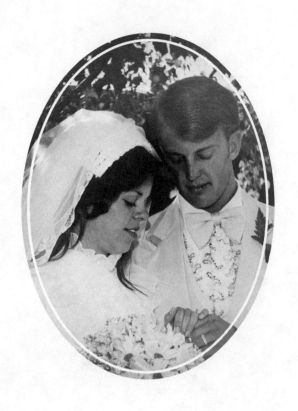

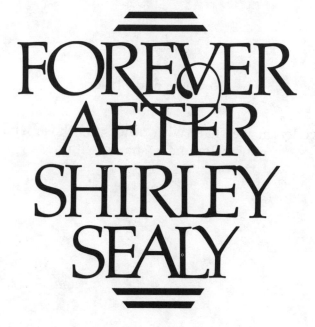

FOREVER AFTER
SHIRLEY SEALY

Deseret Book Company
Salt Lake City, Utah
1979

To Gayle and Skyler

As we learn, we share with others, as those who have
gone before have shared with us.

© 1979 Shirley Sealy
All rights reserved
Printed in the United States of America

Library of Congress Cataloging in Publication Data

Sealy, Shirley.
 Forever after.

  1. Sealy, Gayle Burch. 2. Mormons and
Mormonism—in Utah—Biography. 3. Toxemia of
pregnancy—Biography. 4. Sealy, Devro.
5. Sealy, Shirley. I. Title.
BX8695.S32S42   289.3'3 [B]   79-17933
ISBN 0-87747-779-5

Preface

This is the story of a love that was born, earned, tested, lived, and will endure forever after.

It is with deep humility that I prayerfully try to relate this true story of a valiant young woman who learned the rules and how to keep them. My hope is that this experience might lend insight, courage, and a degree of understanding to others who might also be called upon to endure such trials.

This story is about Gayle Burch Sealy, her husband, Devro, and their son, Skyler. It is written from my own point of view, involving my own feelings and experiences. If it were possible to also include the feelings and emotions of Gayle's family, I'm sure this account would be more effective.

Loving Gayle as I do, I feel it a special pleasure to write her story, and I have tried to express things as Gayle would have expressed them if she were writing this account. She often spoke of her desire to write, and this is my effort and tribute to her.

I thank those whose names are mentioned in the book for their permission to use them. Special gratitude is extended to Jean and Stanley Burch, Gayle's parents. I have purposely stayed away from using more names than absolutely necessary, since I do not wish to involve others or presume to express their feelings. This is Gayle's story, as nearly as I can make it her story. It is the kind of love story the world needs, the kind that contains visible, believable examples of love that can endure forever after.

1

"Not my baby! Not my baby!" I watched Gayle, so young, so full of hurt, try to raise herself up on the hospital bed. Her voice was low and unnatural; her words came in short gasps. The oxygen tube in her mouth would have made talking difficult enough even without the pain. "P-please, don't let them t-take my b-baby."

Darling Gayle. Of course she would protest. Hadn't she always protected herself and her baby ever since she'd known she was going to be a mother? No, even before she'd known: why, she'd been preparing her whole life for this moment. Now, even though the pain was so bad that only a few minutes ago she'd said she wanted to die, she was still protesting anything that might take away her baby's chance for a full life.

Gayle's husband, our son Devro, leaned over his young wife, restraining her tenderly as he kissed her cheek between words: "My Gayle—the doctor says he has to take the baby in order to save your life."

His words were gentle, his arms around her tender, even though his eyes showed the terrible fear tightening around his own heart. He'd always been protective of his bride, prided himself in keeping her beside him. He looked so helpless now.

"No . . . not yet . . . too soon . . ." Her head rolled again and her body knotted into a little ball. He smoothed her hair with his hand, kissed her cheek, her forehead, her small hand, and tried to speak comfort between kisses.

"Don't worry, my Gayle, our baby will be all right. The nurse took me into the nursery and showed me some other little babies born at six months. Some of them do just fine."

"No—" she tried again to protest but couldn't finish what she was trying to say. The words were engulfed by another groan, and her hand tightened on Devro's arm as the pain intensified. Finally her hand slipped off his arm and she was quiet again, except for her labored breathing.

Devro watched her for a few minutes, then got up and began to walk around the room. He reminded me of an animal that had suddenly realized it was trapped inside four walls. He walked around the room as if examining the possibilities of escape, and stopped at the foot of Gayle's bed, his arms stretched forward as he teetered back and forth on the bottom frame of her hospital bed, gazing down at his almost lifeless wife. His face had such a look of desperation, of helpless anxiety; then tenderness appeared as the love he felt showed through his anguish. I watched, wondering what I could say or do to help him. Then Gayle stirred and he instantly came to attention.

"Help me—p-please help me," she pleaded as the pain again twisted her body. Devro's mouth fell open and his eyes widened as her pain clutched at him. It was obviously he was trying hard to understand, but his desperation was frightening, even to me. I stepped close to him and spoke softly.

"She's so frightened, dear; don't let her see that you're frightened too. She needs your strength."

He seemed not to hear, but moved to her side and took her small hand in his own. She hung on to him until the pain eased again and she was quiet. As she relaxed, his head hung down as if he had gone through the same pain, and as he sat there beside her I wondered if he was praying. Yes, I knew instinctively that he was. He'd been prayerful all the days of his life. He was praying, I was praying, we were all praying with all the fervor we'd ever had in praying for anything in our lives. Sweet, beautiful Gayle, with the long, lovely hair. She was an angel already, this daughter-in-law whom I loved as my very own.

2

I looked around the room. It was just an ordinary hospital room, where the nurses came and went, with one exception: beside Gayle, quietly taking care of her needs, sat her mother, Jean. Jean hadn't said much, but it was obvious how concerned she was. Her short hair was in place, her manner calm, and she tried not to show how worried she was. But I knew she was acutely aware of how extremely critical the situation was—more aware than either Devro or I. Jean was a practical nurse and had been beside sickbeds a good many years. She'd seen a lot of illness and knew what signs to look for.

I didn't know Jean very well. I had met her at the wedding about a year ago, and at some of Gayle's showers. But I knew her daughter, my son's wife, and to have a daughter like Gayle, Jean had to be a very special person. I knew also that Dev loved Gayle's parents. He and Jean were close, and I knew he thought Stan, Gayle's father, was a man to seek advice from. Devro and Gayle had a good marriage, had set the right goals, were obedient—so what had happened? Was this real or a nightmare that I'd awaken from? If only it could be a dream!

Only a few hours earlier Gayle had been standing at my back door. She was preparing for her Mutual class to meet at her apartment. It was to be a special evening, and she had prepared refreshments and favors. How she loved those Beehive girls in her ward! They had put her through some moments of concern, and I knew she had spent a lot of time praying about them and about how to teach them what they needed, how to let them know she loved them, so they would feel approved of. Before Mutual that night she and Devro hurried in and out of our home. Then later I had received that strange phone call from Devro.

"Mother?" Devro often said Mother instead of Mom when he was concerned, but now his voice was calm, casual. "Mother, Gayle has a pain."

"Is it bad?"

"Well, I don't know. I think it must be. You know Gayle—she doesn't complain. She was standing there

3

teaching her lesson and suddenly she stopped talking and told me she was a little sick at her stomach—nauseated."

"In the middle of her lesson?"

"Yes. She went on with the story she was telling until she finished it, and then she handed me the book—"

"Do you want me to come down?"

"Would you?"

"Of course. I'm on my way, but call the doctor, huh?"

"All right. The Mutual girls are here but I can take them home."

"I'll hurry. It may be nothing, but . . ."

What had happened next? I tried to think back. I'd gotten in the car and headed for their apartment, only a few blocks away. Dev said he would take the girls home, but as I drove into his driveway he came running out to meet me.

"Mother, will you take the girls home and stop by the ward and tell my Scouts we won't be meeting tonight?"

"Sure. How's Gayle?"

"I called the doctor and he said to bring her right in to the emergency room, just as a precaution. She really hurts."

I asked the girls to get in the car and then ran around to the back of the house to see if I could do anything for Gayle before we left. I met her coming out—she was walking stiffly, and I could tell she didn't want to say anything. Dev followed, still in his work clothes. They were taking off without even a suitcase.

"Mother, tell my Scouts I'll call them tomorrow about getting together, all right?"

"Sure. Don't worry about anything here, I'll take care of—" But he was gone without hearing the last.

Finally the last girl was dropped off, the message was delivered to the Scouts, and I was home calling the hospital. "Dev?"

"Yes, Mom. They think Gayle has toxemia. They want to keep her in the hospital a couple of days to check it out."

A feeling of fear tightened around my heart; I'd heard

of some cases of toxemia. I was frightened and I knew Dev was too, even though his voice was calm. That was the way Dev was, always calm in a crisis. And, after all, this was 1978, and the doctors could do such wonderful things.

No, I wouldn't overreact. I made my voice casual.

"Was she . . . I mean, did she stand the trip all right?"

"Oh, Mom, she was bad. I hit ninety on the way here and hoped I'd find a highway patrolman to clear my way, but I didn't. She scared me."

"Is there anything I can do? Shall I come down?"

"I don't know. It would be nice to have somebody to talk to. Come if you can."

"Shall I call Gayle's mother?"

"Yes, why don't you do that. And her piano students. She's worried about them coming in the morning and not finding her there."

"I'll call them. I think her piano teaching book is here in the piano bench."

I hung up and called Gayle's mother, who lived only a few blocks away, between our home and Gayle's apartment.

"Jean?"

"Yes."

"This is Shirley. I just called the Utah Valley Hospital. Dev took Gayle in. They think she might have toxemia."

After a silence, Jean said, "I just got home from work but I'll go right down."

"Dev wanted you to know."

She thanked me and I hung up, still feeling uneasy. I pulled a medical book out of the bookcase and looked up the entry for toxemia. What I learned didn't make me feel any better. I looked up the piano students while I let my mind race. Gayle had been teaching piano lessons in Dev's old room, which we had turned into a study. I had loved listening to her play the piano while she waited for her students.

I did a few little things around the house, but I was still nervous. Something about this wasn't right. Finally I just junked everything I had to do and got in the car and headed for the hospital.

"Dev, was there any warning of this?" I didn't need to have anybody tell me that Gayle was worse than they had thought.

"Nothing but a little swelling in her feet when we walked around campus at youth conference. You know—you were with her."

"Yes."

"Friday evening when President Kimball spoke, Gayle and I went early so we could get a good seat. Gayle was so excited about the Prophet coming. We got a front row seat and were among the few who shook his hand as he left. Well, anyway, after he talked, while they were setting up for the dance, we went outside and walked around the campus. Her feet were swollen and hot so we found a creek and took off our shoes and put our feet in the cold water, and the swelling went down. Swelling is one of the signs."

"I remember she said that, but I didn't think much of it because my feet were swollen too. Heat and walking often do that normally."

"We didn't worry because she had just been in for her checkup and she was doing just fine."

"I can't understand it. She's always been a good, balanced eater. No junk foods for Gayle. She always wanted to eat things that were good for her baby. Jean," I said, turning to Gayle's mother, who was sitting beside the bed, "did you think there was anything wrong?"

"No. She told me about her feet too, but I didn't think there was any reason for concern. If I had only taken her blood pressure that day, maybe—"

"No warning, just fast."

Gayle moved in her bed again, gasping for air.

"Help me . . . I'm smothering . . ."

That's when Dev ran down the hall and came back with a nurse and some oxygen. After that Gayle rested a while and seemed to be doing better. Everyone was encouraged. After an hour or so, I said, "Dev, I think I'll go home for a while and be on call in case you need anything. Is there anything you need right now?"

He looked down at his work clothes. "I could use a change of clothes."

"I'll get you a change and maybe bring Gayle's robe and slippers for when she gets up, if you want me to."

I drove back to American Fork, picked up the things, delivered them back to the hospital in Provo, and then tried to get Jean to let me take over while she rested.

"I can't rest anywhere yet. I'll just stay here until the crisis is passed," she said.

There was nothing more I could do, so I went home to wrestle with my thoughts and try to sleep.

At about six the next morning our daughter Loni's friends called for a ride to Pep Club. It must have been while they were talking that Dev tried to call home and couldn't get our line, because when I got back from taking the girls to Pep Club, our oldest married daughter, Vicki, called.

"Mother?"

"Yes, Vicki."

"Dev called from the hospital. Gayle has had more complications and they've decided to take the baby."

"Oh, Vicki—"

"Her life is in danger and they think taking the baby will save her."

"Does Dev want me to come?"

"I think he needs both you and Dad. He doesn't want to take you away from anything you have to do, but—"

"Nothing else is important right now. We'll leave right away. Call your sisters, Vicki. They will want to know. And invite them to join us in fasting and prayer. We need their prayers."

"I'll call them. Let us know . . ."

My husband, Milton, and I arrived at the hospital and were directed to the intensive care unit waiting room. We

7

found Devro there, stretched out on a couch, lying in a twisted position as if he had fallen asleep against his will. His face was streaked with tears, and he looked as if he had aged ten years. As we stood there looking down at him, he opened his eyes and sat up. I leaned down and kissed him. Milt sat down beside him and put an arm around his shoulders.

"She's still bad—but they think the baby has a good chance," Dev said. "Oh, I've never prayed so hard in my life."

"We're *all* praying for her," I said as I sat down beside him. He went on talking as if he didn't hear anything but his own words.

"Gayle's a saint already. She's always been a saint. I want her to get well, and our little baby too."

"She'll be blessed, Dev. Heavenly Father has always answered our prayers, and she is worthy."

His head rolled from side to side. "I can't go in there and watch her go through anymore." Even as he was speaking he got up and started down the hall.

"Can't I go in for you, Dev?"

"No, Mom, she might wake up and ask for me or wonder where I am." He took a few steps more, then turned and came back and put his hand out to his father and kissed me. "Thanks for coming—thanks for being here."

"Milt," I said, watching him go, "he's been through so much. Dev hates hospitals."

"He's never been in one since he was born, has he?"

"Oh, for little things, like the time he broke his arm playing football, and the time he ate a poison weed."

"But nothing serious. He's always been so healthy."

"Gayle, too. Those two are nuts about exercise. Why, between the workouts and the karate practice, both of them are strong. How could this happen?"

Milt didn't answer, and I could see that his chin was quivering. He was so tenderhearted where the children and grandchildren were concerned. Looking at him now, it was hard to visualize the hardworking, tough boss who kept everything going for our family. We sat quietly for a while—I was praying again.

Finally I broke the silence. "Milt, you know Dev told me that neither he nor Gayle had ever refused to do anything the other asked. Even that time when Gayle was sick and couldn't do the dishes. Dev said he did them alone, but he was sure in their next house they would have a built-in dishwasher. That's quite a relationship, isn't it?"

Milt nodded. "Gayle can do anything. Remember when the lights went off and I had some little chickens under the brooder? By the time I got home she had found the lantern and had it out in the coop keeping the chickens warm. She's always been thoughtful."

"I wonder how strong they both are? I wonder what they are going to have to face in the next few hours and if—"

Just then a nurse came to tell us there was a phone call for us. I went to answer it.

"Mom?" It was our daughter Linda calling from downstairs. "We're all here. Can we come up?"

"All? You mean all Dev's sisters? Even Judy from Salt Lake?"

"Yes, Vicki called her and she drove down."

"Come up to the waiting room."

There was just time for the girls to see Gayle before the nurse announced that it was time for her to go to surgery. I could see it was helpful to Devro that his sisters were there, and he and his father had been able to give Gayle a blessing. Dev sat with us after they rolled her through the double doors.

"I'd planned on watching this baby born," said Dev, his eyes far away, remembering. "We took one of the classes together and were going to take the rest so I could be with her."

I wanted to help him, to say something that might ease his hurt, but anything I could say he already knew. I looked down at his shoes. He still had his big, heavy work shoes on.

"Dev, we'll have quite a long wait. Would it help you

to freshen up and put on your other clothes?"

He looked at me, a sign that he had heard what I said, and smiled.

"Yeah, Mom, I'd like to do that."

He took the clothes I had brought earlier and went in search of a washroom. As I watched him go I thought how grateful I was for his courage. Dev had always been able to bounce back from every hurt or defeat in his life. How much hurt was there yet to come? Would he still be able to smile and bounce back if anything happened to Gayle or their baby?

2

While we waited for the double doors to open again I sat and thought about these two wonderful kids of ours. I thought about their beginnings and all they had been through together since they met, and even before they met. I didn't know quite as much about Gayle as I did about Devro, though I couldn't have loved her more if I had been her real mother. But Devro . . .

Devro was the fourth child of our five and our only son. What a thrill it had been the day he was born. A son! At last a son, and one with blue eyes and blond hair. Of course, they say all children have blue eyes when they are born, but Devro's were so blue I just knew they would never be any other color.

He had rather large features to be a really good-looking baby, but to me he was handsome. The nurses were afraid of him because his skin was so white. They thought he wasn't normal, but his sister Linda had been that white, so I told them I'd keep him. Then they discovered an unusual heartbeat, and I learned what it was to fight the fear of what I'd do if he didn't live. I had to wait in the hospital for four days while they took tests to make sure he was all right. I called Milt from the hospital when I knew there was danger.

"Don't you think you should come and bless him and give him a name?"

"I'll come and bless him, but we'll name him in church like all of the girls were named."

"But how can you be so confident?"

11

"I have a good feeling about this boy, have had ever since we decided to have him. Don't worry, he'll grow up to be president of the Church or something great like that."

"President of the Church, huh? You sound like a typical father."

"Honey, you just leave this boy to me. All the girls turned out well, didn't they? Well, I left them to you," he laughed. "But this time I know about this boy."

I'd smiled and felt better. And he had been right; we had named the baby Devro in church. The doctors had checked him out and let us take him home, and after a week the funny heartbeat had disappeared.

Had there ever been a baby as loved as Devro? Vicki was fourteen at his birth and turned herself into a second mother. Dev hadn't heard a cross word in connection with himself until after he was two years old. Sometimes he had to cry in his bed, especially on Mondays after a weekend of the whole family spoiling him, but that had been his only discipline. He was easy to handle and easy to love.

A delightful son and plenty of baby tenders—that was our family with Devro. On Sundays I sang in the ward choir, so the family handled him in the congregation. On Relief Society day it was my turn to hold him. He didn't like the nursery, so I let him sit on my lap and look at books as long as he was good. He would sit patiently until the closing prayer was said, and then in his deep voice he would say *"Amen!"* so loudly it would embarrass me. It was funny how he had had that deep masculine voice right from birth, even when he cried. I always thought that was in defiance of my worries about his being feminine with so many sisters.

Dev was always a good actor. At age three he had a part in the roadshow. He and a neighbor girl sang a song, "Wash Up the Dishes, Daddy, Mama's Going to Town," fourteen times in one night. But his acting ability was often wasted in his room when he became too much of a show-off.

Dev had always loved electrical equipment. I would save the old record players, toasters, irons, and anything else that quit running, for him to take apart.

"Throw the stuff out," Milt would say. "I hate all this junk around."

"But he's learning. Can't I throw it away after he takes it apart?"

"What is he learning?"

"Well, for one thing, he's set up a car wash for match-box cars in the basement. He and his friends put it together with some of the electrical stuff they took apart. They charge a penny a wash for all the kids in the neighborhood."

"You don't think he'll get rich, do you?"

"No, but he has the satisfaction of knowing the thing works."

How crazy, I thought, as my mind focused back on the hospital room around me, that I should be reliving his childhood now. But here we were making history again with Devro's child. That's what Dev's life had been—making family history. He and his friends had done a lot of living.

Devro always had a lot of friends, both boys and girls, and his teachers all liked him. He was an individual, that was for sure. One teacher said he wasn't good at art, but when he held his picture up she could always depend on its being the most original. He was that way about what he wore, too. In second grade he had insisted on wearing rolled-up jeans with white socks, tennis shoes, and always an ironed shirt. I thought it was the fad at school and that he was joining the crowd, but when I visited his school I found out he was the only one who dressed that way. Of course, by the next month other children had picked up his fad. And he used to get by on his personality instead of homework. That had been a rough one.

How Dev hated busywork at school. He didn't care about grades and there was nothing I could say or do to make him care. If it hadn't been for Little League football and the help of his coaches, I would never have been able to motivate Devro to get good grades. But the coach required good grades, and what the coach required, Devro did.

My thoughts were interrupted as I looked up to see Dev coming toward us. His clothes were changed, his face washed, and his hair combed. He was smiling. How could he be so cheerful with his insides kicked out? But there he was, smiling his old familiar smile.

"You look good, Master Devro." I used the old family title his sisters had attached to him.

"I feel better too. Everything's going to be all right, Mom."

"Your sisters are still downstairs."

"I'll go talk to them after I find out about Gayle," he said, and went to check with one of the nurses about what was going on.

Devro's sisters each had a special spot in his life. Vicki called him her blue-eyed boy and mothered him. Judy was his constant challenge in sports. She was only four feet ten inches tall, even now when she was the mother of three children, but she was good at all the sports, and she and her boyfriends had constantly given Devro a bad time when he was too boastful. His ego was often choked out of him when he had to compete with Judy. Devro and Linda had become close when she was in college and he was in high school, just before Linda was married. It was Linda who set things right when Gayle was out of town and Devro almost backed out of their engagement. And Loni—Loni was the only girl in our family who had a big brother. He had teased her unmercifully even up to the day he was married. She hated him and adored him both at once.

"Milt," I said, stretching my legs as my memories came to a halt, "I think I'll go down and be with the girls. Will you let me know if anything happens?"

"I'll let you know, Shirl."

The elevator door opened, and I crossed to where the

14

girls sat talking. They looked up as I approached, and I answered the question on their faces before they could ask.

"No word yet. But I'm glad you're here. Dev feels better with all of us around him, I know he does."

"I wondered if we should have gotten Loni out of school and brought her with us," Vicki began.

"No, let her stay. There isn't anything we can do now. She can come tonight. It's a long operation. If the doctors are right, if Gayle reacts as many other cases have done, as soon as they take the baby her condition will turn right around and she'll get better."

"Cute Dev," said Linda, "he's always been the one who's so crazy about children. One of the ladies in our ward said she has watched him strut around ever since he announced Gayle was having a baby. He acts as if he's the one carrying it."

"He's always been crazy about children. He used to come home and tell me he'd fallen in love—so seriously—and it always turned out to be some little four- or five-year-old girl he had seen."

"Is he alone up there now?"

"No. Jean and your father are with him."

"How is Dad taking this?"

"He's finding it hard to fight the tears, Judy. You know how tenderhearted he is. He loves Gayle so much, just like you girls. As soon as she's out of the operating room, he's going to work. You know your father— working is his way of getting a grip on his emotions."

"Those kids are really loved," said Vicki. "I can't believe how many people are calling and offering prayers."

As we sat there talking, more relatives began to come: my sisters and their husbands, Dev's cousins and friends. The waiting room on the first floor began to fill up, and how it helped! We were a close family, and we needed each other in times of crisis.

I went back upstairs to tell Dev how many had come, but he was busy talking to Jean, so I sat down and talked to Milt.

"Milt, I wonder what is ahead for Dev and Gayle."

"His life is going to be changed no matter what happens in that surgery."

"If only the baby will breathe—at least then they will know they have a baby and will be able to raise it sometime."

"Losing a baby will be hard on Gayle. She has planned for so long."

"Remember how excited she was when Santa Claus made their announcement at Christmas?"

"I remember how embarrassed Gayle was that Dev talked about it so boldly."

"But she was happy and proud that Dev wanted everyone to know."

"You would think he would break under a strain like this, Mom. I would. Look at me now—all I can do is cry."

"But when you are the one facing the problem, you hold up just as he is doing."

As if in answer, Dev came down the hall, sat down by us, and put his arm around my shoulders.

"Mom, it's going to be all right."

"If you say so," I smiled. "You are a pretty stubborn boy when you make up your mind."

"What do you mean?"

"I've just been thinking back over your life, and a minute ago I was remembering the time when you were a little guy in Primary and you wouldn't sing. You made up your mind you weren't going to sing, and nothing the chorister could say would make you sing. When I inquired why you were putting your teacher through this, you said you weren't going to sing again until you got your guitar."

Dev laughed and I went on. "Well, that was the first time we ever heard that you wanted a guitar."

"But Dad got me one."

"Yes, he did, and you still wouldn't sing until you and Paul did that little concert in the basement together. That was such fun. You made up the songs, set the stage, and rigged up that stand that looked like a mike, and sent out invitations."

"Bob plunked out all those invitations with one finger on your typewriter."

"And forgot to put on the date. You wondered why you didn't have a big crowd. Were you about ten years old then?"

"About that."

"Then came the drums. One concert and a couple of songs in public and you were ready for the drums."

"And you made me earn them. I practiced for a whole year on a drum pad first. I hated that drum pad."

"But you did it and took piano lessons from Linda too. Remember, that was part of the deal to earn your drums, that you take basic piano."

"How I remember!"

"You took a lesson every Saturday until you passed off the first book, and we didn't find out until after you had your drums that you'd learned that whole book by rote and couldn't read a note of music."

"What made you think of that, Mom?"

"Remembering how stubborn you are when you make up your mind."

Small talk, anything to fill the gaps; memories, so unimportant in comparison to what was going on in surgery. But memories were important too. "To predict the future, examine the past." This was a motto I lived by. And what was Dev's past? What was Gayle's past?

For one thing, Dev had a good background in church activity. He was always good to go to his meetings, though once there was a time when he almost quit Primary. The teacher had assigned each of the children a secret friend, and Dev's secret assignment was a girl he didn't like. She was a good girl and we loved her family, but she was forward, and Dev didn't like forward girls.

"I won't do it," he said stubbornly. "I won't have her for a secret friend."

"Are you sure you know what it means to be a secret friend?"

"I won't talk with her or play with her or—"

"You don't have to do that. Just be nice to her and say hello when you pass, and think kind thoughts about her, and whenever any of the other kids say bad things you try to say something nice instead. She doesn't have to know—that's what secret means. You just have to be a friend and think kindly of her in your heart."

"Well, I guess I can do that."

I watched him after that and I never did hear him say anything against her again. That was Dev—when he made up his own mind he followed through. It was inspiring him to make up his mind that was difficult for me.

When Dev started Mutual we had another difficult time. Mutual came on Little League night. He could make it to opening exercises if he hurried when the practice was over. The first night he did make it, but the second night he was late, and the third week he just stayed for a few extra plays with Kevin on purpose.

"Dev, you were too late for Mutual."

"I don't like Mutual, Mom. We don't do anything, and the Scoutmaster is stupid."

"Stupid or not, he has been called to be your leader and your place is there."

End of discussion. Dev had a way of turning me off when he didn't want to hear. The next week when he was late again, he arrived home to find me almost ready to leave.

"Where you going, Mom?"

"I'm going to Mutual and I'll be going every Mutual night, so you will have to get home in time to tend Loni. I can't be late, so you will have to hurry. I hope I don't have to talk to your coach about letting you leave a few minutes early."

"I don't want to tend Loni."

"I know, but I don't always want to wash the shirts that you wear either. We all have to do some things we don't want to do. I'll make a deal with you: If you'll get home on time and tend Loni, then I'll wash your football clothes for you."

"What if I want to go to Mutual?"

"If you so desire, I guess I'll have to let you go, since you have been invited, but you can't go once and not the next time and keep your teacher worrying about you. You have to decide to go or to tend Loni so I can go."

"I want to go to Mutual."

"You're too late for tonight."

"I'll hurry. I'll make it in time for class."

That one was conquered. He had grasped the concept and Mutual was never really a problem anymore, even though there were times when he had to make choices about it. Making choices—that was what built character. Had he learned enough to accept whatever would come out of those double doors?

Going to church was more than just a habit for Dev. He had a natural, deep sense of justice and seemed to have been born with a love of truth. When he was baptized we had one of our special talks and I tried to explain how the Holy Ghost works and the power that comes with that gift. Dev was impressed, and the next morning I knew something had hit him because at breakfast he said, "Mom, that was neat, what we talked about last night. Can we talk about that again?"

Yes, I thought, looking at the closed double doors that would surely open any minute now—Dev had handled each step in his life as well as could be expected for his background and teachings. I was proud of him. I could say that and really mean it. He would make a good father, he was a sweet loving husband, and he had always been an obedient son. "Please, Heavenly Father, bless him now," I pleaded quietly. "Bless him now as thou hast done in the past. Whatever he has to face, let him retain that goodness he has always had and let him be worthy of a wife like Gayle. Bless their lives and their marriage and their baby—please, Heavenly Father."

3

"Mr. Sealy." A nurse appeared and we all came to attention. "The operation is over and your wife will be coming out of surgery soon. If you and your parents would like to catch a glimpse of your baby, the doctor will be coming right down this hall in just a few seconds."

"My baby! I'm a father!" Dev's smile broadened, covering his whole face. "I'm a father. Nurse, is—"

"The baby is alive. I don't know any details, but the doctor will be here to talk to you soon."

"What do you think, Dev?" I asked. "A girl or a boy?"

He grinned some more. "Gayle thought we were having a girl. I like little girls—but a man always wants a son—oh, I don't know."

Just then the nurse appeared again to tell us there was a phone call. I went to answer it. My sister, terribly worried, was calling from Salt Lake City. When I got back the baby had already come through the double doors, and I saw only Dev's back as he followed the doctor into the nursery. "A boy," said Jean excitedly, her tiredness momentarily disappearing. "They have a son."

"A son! Devro has a son! Won't Gayle be surprised?"

"And thrilled," said Jean. "Our first grandson on the Burch side."

More small talk—for a while we put a lot of it together while we waited, and then Dev appeared again. His shoulders seemed a little straighter and the old football walk was a bit more brisk.

"He weighs three pounds four ounces. Not bad for a little six-month boy, is it?"

"Not bad at all. How does he look, Dev?"

"He looks great. The doctor thinks he has a pretty good chance. You should see the equipment they have in that nursery. My son is on an open incubator. He has his own waterbed. He's so cute."

"Does he look like you?"

"Sure does, but like Gayle too, around his mouth."

"Blond hair?"

"Blond hair and blue eyes. He has big shoulders and the tiniest hips and bottom you ever saw. He's a cute little baby."

"Can I tell your sisters or do you want to?"

"Go ahead, Mom. I want to be here when Gayle comes out."

I left then to ring for the elevator, but I heard Dev say to his father, "Come and see him, Dad. We can look through the window while the doctor finishes his examination."

In the next hour there was a parade of family members peeking, one at a time, through the tiny window while Dev, inside, with a sterile gown on, would lift up a little foot or a hand. The tiredness in his face disappeared as he assumed his new role as a father.

It took the doctors a while to finish up before they finally rolled Gayle into the recovery room. I heard one doctor say, as she was wheeled past him, "That was difficult."

Later, when we knew Gayle was recovering in her room, Milt left to go to work. And since Gayle was still asleep, Dev went with his sisters to get something to eat. When they came back I decided to go home for a while.

"I'll stay if you need me, Dev."

"No, Mom, you go ahead. We'll be all right. Gayle is already half-awake. I told her about our son and she nodded and mumbled something. She's happy."

I kissed Dev, and as he put his arms around me and thanked me for being there he said, "He's a cute little boy. If only he can live for Gayle to see him when she is better."

My daughters and I climbed in the car and started for home with Vicki at the wheel. Members of the family who had gathered had all dispersed when the baby was born. For the moment the crisis seemed to have passed. The girls were full of chatter.

"Dev was so cute at lunch," said Linda, her voice full of emotion. "He said over and over how cute his little son was, and then he said he guessed he didn't have much of a chance to live, but that it would be so nice if he could." As she spoke the tears rolled down her face.

"Our little brother is so strong," said Vicki, her chin quivering as she struggled to watch the traffic. "He's taking everything so well. His attitude is so tender and obedient that it just hurts my heart."

"And he's even cheerful," added Judy. "I don't see how he does it. He was smiling and joking with us, remembering things Gayle said."

"He's been through so much," said Linda. "I hope Gayle comes out of this fast. He needs her so much."

"I'm glad she's out of pain. She went through so much because the doctors didn't want to give her too much medication. They wanted the baby to have every chance. Now at least she can have some painkillers if she needs them."

"And maybe Dev can get some rest now, too."

"It's really helped him to have all of you there," I said. "I'm so glad we have each other, girls; it would be hard to go through things like this alone." I stopped talking as a thought occurred to me.

"Mother?" Vicki inquired. She always seemed so sensitive to my thoughts. "Mother, what's the matter?"

"I was just thinking. The baby isn't out of danger yet. If anything happens, it would be terrible if Dev were there without..."

"Do you want to go back?"

"I think I should. You don't mind? I should have brought my own car."

"We're only a few blocks away. I'll just turn around and take you back. Richard and I will come back this evening and then you can come home."

"All right. Your father will be back by then, too."

I went back to the hospital to talk and wait, to try to sleep sitting up, to read and pray, and to answer phone calls that came to the hospital for the family. The day wore on.

We knew Gayle's doctors had called a specialist to go over her condition. When he finished his examination he asked that we come together to meet with him. So there we stood, Devro, Jean, and I, and the doctor faced us, his expression serious. I couldn't believe what he was saying, yet his words were too serious for doubt.

"I want you to know," he said, looking directly at us, "that there isn't anyone in this hospital tonight whose condition is any more critical than your wife's, Mr. Sealy. Do you understand?"

He waited and Dev nodded as he repeated, "I understand."

Then the doctor told us everything he had found wrong: how very ill Gayle was, that all her vital organs were involved, that taking the baby hadn't made her condition turn around as they had expected. Yes, there was some hope, but nothing really definite. It would depend on what the next few hours brought, and how she responded to treatment. Maybe by morning there would be some change, but right now saying that she had a fifty-fifty chance was an exaggeration.

I stood there thinking, *Gayle might die? How can that be? No, not after all she's been through!*

Somehow the doctor finished talking and left us. We stood there a moment in a daze; then Jean went into Gayle's room, and Dev started walking. I went with him. He took my hand and we walked back and forth a little. Someone stopped us to ask about Gayle; Dev answered something and then he pulled me down the hall with him toward a room at the end of the intensive care section where he had rested a little the night before. Once we were inside, he fell apart.

"Not my Gayle—not my Gayle! Why? Why?" His harsh sobs tore at me. I swallowed the anguish inside myself as I tried to find something to say that might help him.

"I don't know, Dev. I don't know. I wish I did, but I don't."

"What will I do? How will I live without her?"

My mind raced as I listened, knowing he was being ripped apart inside. He had been so strong and brave, so cheerful through it all, so comforting to everyone else around who needed help. Now he himself had to have some help, and I was so helpless. I had thought perhaps the baby might die, but not Gayle too. Not Gayle. But the doctor's words were burning inside me. He had been trying to prepare us.

"Not my Gayle, Heavenly Father," Dev cried. "I need her; I can't live without her."

In answer to his pleading voice I heard myself saying, "You won't have to live without her, Dev."

He looked at me incredulously, as if he wanted me to prove my words, to give him anything he could cling to. I hurried on, not even sure of what I was saying, as if the words weren't coming from me.

"Dev, you married Gayle in the temple for time and all eternity. You won't ever have to be without her unless you don't live worthy of her. She is yours forever and ever."

"I know, Mother, I know." His response gave me some hope that he was comforted. It was all he had to hold on to, and he grasped it like a drowning man. I kept talking. He already knew anything I could say—he knew more than I did—but we needed the sound of the words right then.

"The worst that can happen, Dev, is that she might have to go on ahead, but the time won't be long. The millennium is so close even if she does go—and she hasn't gone yet."

"That's right. It isn't very far off, is it? Oh, Mother, I can't let her go. She isn't going to die, Mother. She isn't..."

"Dev, if Heavenly Father has a greater mission for her, you wouldn't keep her here, would you?"

"No, Mother, I wouldn't do that." He spoke firmly, as if he were annoyed that I would even ask. I wanted to cry, to sob, to hug and comfort him, to show him how proud I was to have a son like him, a daughter like Gayle. But I couldn't cry now—not now. He was having a hard enough time without my letting down. He didn't need my sympathy; he needed strength. Besides, I knew that if I started crying now I couldn't stop. I watched as Dev got hold of himself.

"Who is here, Mom?"

"You mean downstairs?"

"Yes. Who is here?"

"Whom do you want? Vicki and Richard are coming, and your father. Whom do you want?"

"I want everybody. Call Vicki and Richard, Linda and Dale, Judy and Neal, Uncle Andy, Dad, and Kevin—get Kevin . . ." He was fighting now, and I could tell he didn't want to fight alone.

"Do you want me to call the bishop?"

"Yes, call him."

"I called him this morning and he said he was coming tonight, but I'll call again."

"Call them, Mother. I don't want to be alone. I've got to go to Gayle now, but get the family here."

As I dialed and waited, in my mind's eye I could see Dev trying to pull himself together to go in and see his wife. He wouldn't let her see his grief or his fear, I knew. He had come this far with faith and a sweet spirit of humility and confidence in his Heavenly Father, the same way he had faced everything on his mission. He would stand it all; he would be all right as long as he had Gayle, but what would he do if she . . . but she wasn't gone, not yet, and the doctor had said there was a chance. A chance was all she needed. We weren't trying to do anything against the will of our Heavenly Father. We had prayed for what was best for her and the baby and Dev. We had asked that she be healed; we weren't trying to tell Heavenly Father how to heal her or how to answer our prayers. "Thy will be done—" that was always the way Dev prayed. We just wanted our Father's attention.

"Hello, Linda?"

"Mother? You sound terrible. What's the matter?"

"Oh, Linda, Gayle is so sick. Call Dad, find him if you can, and tell the girls. Tell Loni we need her prayers. I'll call the bishop from here."

"Mother, I thought she was going to be all right."

"That's what we all thought. Oh, pray, dear, pray— and Dev needs us here. There is so much wrong."

I called and talked and called and talked and waited and prayed—and then they came. Those we called came, and those who cared and heard came, and Gayle's family came; the waiting room filled up as the hospital settled down for the night. As people came we prayed separately and as a group. Gayle was given another blessing... and we waited.

In Gayle's room another drama was taking place. Because of the oxygen tube she couldn't talk very well, but she could make Dev understand. When he stooped to kiss her face, she leaned toward him, responding to his touch even in her discomfort and fear. He told her about the baby and she was happy. He talked to her about a name and together they decided not to wait until she could see him, but to name him immediately, just in case.

"Devro Skyler," she whispered hoarsely.

"Devro Skyler," Dev repeated. "All right, my Gayle, I'll go with the bishop and we'll name him now."

So Devro's son, Gayle's son, was named as he lay on his hospital waterbed with the latest equipment monitoring his progress. Then the vigil started. It was a vigil that lasted into the early morning hours with Dev going from Gayle's room to Skyler's nursery and back again. While he covered that trek, I went from the main lobby to the intensive care lobby to take messages back and forth and to answer calls. Again I was a living part of the elevator that went up and down, an elevator that clanged and stopped and clanged and started again while the family held together and prayed and prayed and couldn't do anything but let Dev know they were there.

At about two in the morning Devro came down to the lobby to make a speech. He smiled at all his loved ones who had come to be with him, and his strong spirit of faith and trust came through to us all.

"I want to thank you all for coming. Believe me, I need your strength. I can't tell you how I appreciate you. Gayle has taken a turn for the better. Just now, the doctor has reported that things look a little better. So I think you can all go home and get some sleep. I love you all so very much and I thank you from my heart."

He stayed with us then for a little while, going from one to another to talk and give his thanks and to say good-bye as they left. I stayed another hour or so and then drove home. Home to think and to try in vain to sleep. I needed sleep so I could be of more help if I was needed, but sleep was a long way from my thoughts. Finally my body, exhausted from the ordeal of two days, took over my mind and I slumped onto my bed, still praying.

4

*U*nable to sleep more than a couple of hours, I got up to view the sky as the early morning light began to show from behind the silhouetted mountains above our home. Devro loved those mountains, and he had used them many times in his life as a refuge, a secret place to climb, to sit and think his problems into solutions. These were the mountains he had tramped with his dog, Ky. They were the mountains he had missed on his mission and the mountains he had climbed when he had had to battle the decision about his marriage. He had even run away to these mountains once in his youth. There had been a heated discussion between Dev and me over something I couldn't even remember now, and he was going out on his own. How well I remembered what I said to him as he packed.

"Fine, Dev, if you want to try living on your own. I think a boy should get out into the world and see what it's like out there. If you think that will be easier than living a few simple rules, you deserve the right to find out. When you go, Devro, I won't even try to stop you, but I will get down on my knees and stay on my knees pleading with the Lord to teach you what you need to know fast, so you can return quickly before you become hardened by problems that might slow you down in your progress. I'll never quit praying until you return, Devro."

He took his dog and went up those very mountains for about half a day, coming home the happy Devro we all knew and loved.

Read the past to foresee the future, I repeated in my

mind. What was their future? What would tomorrow bring for Dev, Gayle, and Skyler?

There beside me, in the bookcase Dev had built, was his book of remembrance, and Gayle's next to it. I took the books down and opened Dev's. I didn't know why; I didn't really expect to find any answers, but my thoughts were so completely with him and Gayle that it seemed as if it would help to remember them when they were so young, so full of the future. So much had happened to them both in such a short time. How much could they take? Hurts, hits, fun, and fast living—that had always been the motto of our family. Get as much accomplished in as short a time as possible. Put our whole family together, and the things we had asked for, and there was a lifetime of miracles piled up. We had always been very blessed. Especially Devro.

Back . . . back to the time we had moved to Highland. That was a whole year before he met Gayle.

Devro Sealy hit the football field of American Fork High School early in the morning in the late summer before his sophomore year. He was going out for quarterback. If the coach couldn't fit him into that position he meant to show him he was the hardest hitter on the team and end up on defense. Dev always dreamed big and fought hard. He believed the motto his coach had drummed into him: "Winning isn't everything; winning is the only thing." And he got the quarterback position in his sophomore year.

If told in detail, Devro's football life would fill a book. He loved the game, dreaded the long, strenuous practices, fought the rules, and learned to live by them. The challenges he faced, the victories and disappointments, the faith he had in his coaches, the shaking of that faith and its restoration—all were part of playing football for Devro. The fight to keep his position on the team in his second and third years was a tough one. One night as he left for practice he sort of mumbled under his breath, "I'm not taking any more. I'm going to knock those two guys out and get them out of my way. They know I'm a hard hitter and I can put them right out."

"What if you hit one of them just right—just hard enough—and kill him?"

"Mom! Other guys keep their positions by knocking the other guy out."

"But what if—"

"But I won't! Mother, I just don't want to fool around anymore. This is my year to play football. I've worked hard all summer and I'm going to keep my position."

"All right. You have to live with yourself."

"Other guys do it."

"But you aren't other guys, you are Dev Sealy, and you live by the laws of justice."

"You always say that, and you think it will stop me. I have to do what I have to do."

"Go ahead. I'm not afraid. You've always chosen well in the past—I'm not going to lose faith in you now."

"Mother!"

He opened the door and was gone. When he returned later I said, "Well?"

Dev shook his head. "I couldn't do it. Those guys are my friends."

There were times when Dev wanted to quit football and never play again. Other times he lived, breathed, ate, and scheduled his whole life around the game. Once, when my husband couldn't attend an important game, he asked Dev if he could give him a blessing. Dev was a little hesitant—he didn't want to misuse the power of prayer—but after a minute he decided to have the blessing. His father blessed him to make right decisions for his life and to be an example of the gospel for his team. Then he left for work and Dev left for school.

Dev's team lost the game that day. He hadn't had an opportunity to do what they had planned or what he felt he could do. This was it, I decided. Dev would quit. He had been undecided about the whole thing lately, and I felt this was the time. But to my surprise, when I got home he was feeling great.

"Are you going to give up football now, Dev?"

"No, Mother," he said, putting his arm around me. "I'm part of that ball team and I'm going to stay even if all they want me to do is carry the water jug."

Those were rough days. When I saw his ability, saw what he could do and what he had given up for the game, and then saw things that a lot of people recognized as being obviously unjust, sometimes I would steam inside. But Dev would say, "You won't say anything, will you, Mother?"

"I'm part of the crowd. I can have an opinion; I pay for my ticket."

"But you won't say anything, will you, Mother?"

"Other people do."

"But you're my mother, so I know you won't."

Dev had a lot of successes in football. He loved playing defense and hitting. He loved passing the ball, and he practiced and practiced and practiced. Sometimes I went into his room at night to see if he had enough quilts over him, and there he would be, his eyes closed, passing the football in his sleep. The record he made that year, of passing the longest distance football, he earned half in his waking hours and half in his sleep.

Dev learned more from his football experience than how to play the game. He learned to develop his own character. He learned to give and take under pressure, to be tough but kind, to handle the panic of those hours before the gun went off—so many truths of life. Later he wrote home from his mission, "Everything I go through out here I can relate to what I learned in football."

Football was not Dev's only interest at this time, however. He had the normal emotions toward girls and always enjoyed the company of the fairer sex. Being an only son in a family with four girls, he had a lot of practice handling woman talk, but one afternoon, shortly after he started high school, he said, "Mom, I want to talk to you about girls."

"About girls?"

"Yes. I want to know how you can keep a girl a friend, date her, and still have her around when and if you want to marry her."

"You mean you don't want to get serious or have to break up?" He nodded and I went on, "Well, as my mother told me, once he has kissed you he isn't content anymore just to hold your hand. If you stick to holding hands and doing fun things instead of getting emotionally involved, you can go with a girl for a long time. Once you get into the emotional attachment, it's either get married—too young—or break up. Build friendships, do crazy things, and then let romance come along when you decide it is time for marriage."

"No making out?"

"I'm not trying to tell you it isn't great. I hope you will be the kissingest husband a girl ever had, but when you are trying to decide which girl you want to marry, stay away from emotion. If you never do anything with a girl that you can't do in front of everybody, you won't have any regrets. You won't feel guilty or embarrassed or obligated. So many relationships are based on obligation—and that's a poor foundation for love and romance."

"I get it—I think."

Dev took seminary in high school. It was in there, in his junior year, that he met Gayle. The two of them had told me about it often enough, but the account in Gayle's journal gave full details:

"In our seminary class, the class president was a good-looking quarterback who seemed to be stuck on himself. He was always kind to me but he liked to tease me. I didn't like him very much because of his teasing. But deep down inside I know I loved every minute of his teasing. I always hoped he would take an interest in me, but a so-called complex led me to think that I wasn't good enough to ever go on a date with him.

"In September of my sophomore year, one day I was walking down the hall when Devro Sealy, the good-looking quarterback, came up to me and asked me if I would go to the Sophomore Slide with him. This was such a surprise to me that I thought it was a joke for him and his friends to laugh at. Especially when the Sophomore Slide wasn't until March. I felt so bad that he would play a trick on me that I told him I would have to talk to my Mom about it. It was my way out so I wouldn't get hurt. Well, I didn't see him for about a week after that; he didn't talk to me or even look at me. I felt really bad, so I decided to walk up to him and ask him if his offer was still good. I did it and he told me that he still wanted to take me. We even went out to a couple of shows before the dance came around. He didn't act very interested in me, but he always said hello to me and treated me very well. . . .

"These feelings may seem meaningless to whoever reads this, but the experience with Dev made me make a big change in my life. My attitude about myself changed completely. I had one hundred times more confidence in myself. I felt like really getting involved in every kind of school and church activity.

"My first attempt at getting involved was trying out for Pep Club. They did marches at the halftime of games and participated in competitions. My older sisters had both been members, so I wanted to follow in their footsteps. I always had and still do have a very high opinion of them both. However, this attempt was a failure. I did not make it in. All my friends who made it told me that they thought that I didn't make it because I had to miss all the morning practices for early morning seminary. But I knew the only reason I didn't make it was that I just didn't try hard enough. I didn't put forth enough effort.

"I was hurt, but I quickly got over it. I knew that I would try again next year but when I did, I would make sure I was ready and I knew I would make it.

"School started again and I was now a junior. I was uninvolved and this made me feel useless. I tried out for a part in the school play but I didn't get the part I wanted because I was too shy to really put my heart into acting, and I couldn't sing very well—mostly because I didn't have enough confidence in myself. I worked hard at school and tried to get ready for Pep Club tryouts again the following spring. I was determined I would make it this time. I worked hard attending all the practices, getting in shape to get down in the splits, and doing everything possible to make me do well on the tryout days. The tryout was very successful, and I felt I had made it into the club.

"The next morning I was awakened by three girls squirting sugar water at me. They took me in my pajamas and initiated me all morning from 6 A.M. until school started. . . ."

The morning sun was just beginning to warm the front room now. I closed Gayle's journal and slipped it and Dev's book back onto the shelf. What a fighter our little Gayle was! Suddenly I wanted to read more about her life, to know more about her, about what had happened in her life before I knew her. I had met her while she was going through those things she had written about, but Dev had been out with her only a few times. He was still going with other girls then. Dev had always had a lot of girls, but he never went with any that I didn't like. He was pretty choosy. When was it he first began to be serious about Gayle? Oh, not until—my thoughts were interrupted by the sudden ringing of the telephone. Fear tightened around my heart. Would that be Dev? Was there anything wrong? Loni appeared in the doorway.

"Mom, the phone is for you. Dev is calling from the hospital."

5

"Mom?"

"Yes, Dev. How is Gayle?"

"About the same. She isn't good. Her father came last night and we gave her another blessing."

"The ward has started a fast; did I tell you?"

"I talked to the bishopric last night—or was it this morning? They said both wards are joining together. I appreciate that."

"Is the baby all right? How's little Skyler?"

"He's so cute, Mom. I talked to him this morning and he opens his eyes wide when I talk to him. He's a good little boy. I told Gayle all about him. Gayle's thirsty today, but they won't let her drink yet. She was trying to get the nurses to give her a real drink of water and not just swab her mouth. I was out a minute and when I came back in, the nurse told me she wanted a chocolate Coke."

"A chocolate Coke?"

"Yeah, you know how funny that is: she has never had a Coke in her life and she doesn't eat chocolate. I told them she must be mad at them. You know Gayle has a temper when she gets upset. I guess she was giving them a bad time . . . thirsty enough to have a chocolate Coke!" He laughed, then went on. "Mom, are you coming to the hospital today?"

"I'm on my way, if you need me."

"I just thought you could bring me a change of clothes—or maybe I can get away later when Jean gets back. She went home to shower. I don't want to leave Gayle, but I do need a shower."

"I can come down and stay while you come home, or I can bring you some things. I thought I would go to the temple and put Gayle's name in, and Skyler's. I thought going through the temple would—"

"That's great, Mom. Why don't you pick up some clothes at our apartment on your way there?"

"I'll be there right away."

"And Mom?"

"Yes."

"Can you cash a check for me and bring me some money? I want to take some of Gayle's family to breakfast and I'm out of cash."

"Sure, dear. I'll hurry. I'll bet you're beginning to worry about the high cost of hospitals right now."

"Yeah, I thought maybe I would be here scrubbing floors the rest of my life. But I've been talking to the nurses and there's help, they tell me."

"Dad says maybe your insurance covers some of this. He's checking into that today. The main thing is just to get Gayle and Skyler well."

"I can do anything if I can just get my family out of the hospital."

"Right. I'll pray for that. See you as soon as I can."

"Hurry, Mom, I would like to pay for breakfast."

I hung up the phone, raced to the shower, then ran to the kitchen to squeeze fresh juice and get the family on their way. I was almost ready to leave when the phone began to ring. Four calls, one after another, came before I could make it to the door. Everyone was so concerned; everyone wanted to help somehow, to do something.

I burst into the hospital just as Gayle's family and Dev were finishing breakfast; they had been too hungry to wait. I slipped the cash into Dev's hand, feeling guilty for being so slow. Then we went upstairs to see Gayle and Skyler.

Gayle didn't look good. I was frightened when I saw her, even more than I had been the night before, but Dev was cheerful and his courage helped me. Skyler looked better. They had put him on oxygen too.

"His lungs aren't as developed as they should be," explained Dev. "They expected that, of course. He can breathe on his own, but the oxygen helps save his strength. I rub his little feet and exercise him. Sometimes I put my finger in his hand, and he really has a grip."

"How many times a night do you go in to see Skyler?"

"Whenever the doctors kick me out of Gayle's room. The nurses let me scrub and put on a gown, and I go in and talk to my son."

We were standing in the hall outside the intensive care room where Gayle was. The nurse came to the door and told Dev he could come in for a minute. I waited and watched as he walked boldly in with a smile on his face, leaned over his wife's bed, and kissed her cheek, her forehead, and her hand. Her lips were dry and her mouth full of the oxygen pipe, but she responded to his touch with a move of her head and a squeeze, limp as it was, of her hand. She was so young, so lovely—and so very ill. I wondered if Devro knew how ill she was, and then knew the thought was foolish. Of course he knew, but he was treating her as he always had, not brooding or talking sick.

I stood there until the doctor came and asked Devro to leave again. They were checking her very closely; a nurse was with her constantly, and specialists came frequently. Dev came out and put his arm around me, and we started to walk toward the elevator. On the way he stopped twice to comfort others—a woman waiting for word of her son, someone else's relatives—he stopped to inquire and to give some comforting words. At the elevator I tightened my grip on his arm.

"Bless you, Devro. You have such strength—if Gayle can just lean on you . . ."

"It will be all right, Mother."

"I know. Kiss Skyler for me, and tell Gayle I love her."

"I will, Mother."

On the way to the temple I was thinking about Dev's life again. It seemed like such a little while since he had graduated from high school. He wasn't really excited about the graduation exercises or the dance that followed. That was Dev, though: he filled the requirements but didn't care about the papers. The real fun came after graduation, when he and two of his friends continued the family custom of going to Bear Lake to celebrate. They had a ball at Bear Lake for three days and came back with homemade haircuts, missionary style. They were all planning missions and would get their calls within the following year.

It was crazy, thinking back to the fun times, when the drama of real life was going on in the hospital. But it helped to think back, to remember when Dev and Gayle were just beginning the steps that would lead them to marriage.

Dev had started a fencing business in high school, and following graduation he worked it full time. I was worried that he wouldn't make enough money to get to the university. I wanted him to have one term at BYU while he waited for his mission call. It was important to me that he have the experience of college before he went away. Then the freshman fears would be over, and it would be easier for him to go back and finish after his mission.

"Dev, I admire you for starting a business and wanting to be independent. But I feel that this isn't the time for you to be fussing around with this fencing business when you could be making good money working with your father."

"Don't worry, Mom. I'll make the money for college and my mission, or I won't go."

"That's what worries me. I know how independent you are, and I'm afraid you will wait until there isn't enough time left to register."

"I told you I'll make it."

"I believe you, Dev, but I'm going to do a lot of praying just the same."

He worked hard at his fencing business, and I had to admit that he put up some good-looking fences without any help from his father or me. He put the money he made back into equipment for the business. That was all right; it wasn't hard for Devro to give up clothes and spending money. He had been used to that when he gave up potential summer jobs so he could play football. But as registration came closer, I began to panic. When his fences were all up, he figured his expenses and profits, and that night he said to his father, "I'm going broke, Dad. I could make this business go if I had more time. I know I can make it go when I get home, but right now I'm going broke. Do you think I can get a job installing doors with your company?"

"Why not try? You have learned how to install from me and you do a good job. Why don't you run in and ask the company boss?"

So he did. Dev pledged himself to the company and was hired; then suddenly he was flying all over the United States alone, and to save his expense money, he slept on the floors of churches where he installed the doors. Sometimes he worked around the clock until time to come home. But he made enough money to get into college. I remember how proud I was the morning he drove down to Brigham Young Univerity with his briefcase by his side. My son, enrolled at BYU. I loved the idea.

Memories . . . yes, but now was now and we had new problems to face. In the past when I had had problems I had gone to the temple just to enjoy the calmness of that atmosphere, and to do something for somebody else instead of worrying about myself. Then I would go home and go about doing the things I had to do, and somehow I would be guided to make the right decision or to say the right things, or sometimes I would just be inspired to change my attitude toward the problem. I didn't expect that going to the temple would solve my problems, but it seemed to give me strength and help and more knowledge—all of which made it easier to cope with my difficulties calmly. I needed that calmness now; I needed to feel close to my Heavenly Father, and the temple was the closest place to heaven that I knew of on this earth.

I was sleepy during the session. Not having had sleep for two nights, I expected that. The quiet atmosphere relaxed me, but even though my eyes were heavy, there seemed to be new meaning in the words I had heard so often. When the session was over and I gathered up my things, preparing to leave, I felt better, lifted somehow. I hadn't had any visions or personal revelations of what was going to happen, but I knew that Skyler, Gayle, and Dev were being blessed, and that whatever happened would be all right.

I hadn't had time to prepare for my speaking engagement that afternoon, but I prayed hard, and the Lord helped me through it all right. Then it was back to the hospital again for a few hours, and finally home to wash some clothes for Dev—the only help I could give him right then. Even when I was finally home, my mind was still in the hospital. I couldn't sleep, so I picked up Gayle's book again. Her words, written in her own hand, seemed to leap out and make her sound alive and well again.

"The summer after I made it into Pep Club was spent in early morning practices. I also started karate lessons. Devro talked me into taking karate. He believes that every woman should be able to defend herself and her children. This philosophy hit me hard, and I felt that I would like to be able to defend my children if they were ever attacked. I worked hard and really hated it at first, mainly because I kept getting hurt, but Dev kept prodding me on. I went out with him often now, but I wouldn't let myself get excited because I thought I would get hurt. He was very kind to me and I grew to love him dearly. We did many things together during my senior year—things such as jogging, practicing karate, going to church, watching TV, and hiking. We both loved to hike. That Christmas he surprised me with a gift that was the best thing that could have happened to me at that time. It was a necklace with a small cultured pearl on it. From then on Dev took me out quite steadily, and I grew to love him as I had never loved a man before. He would pick me up at school and we would go over to the indoor track at the BYU. This is the one thing I really admired about Dev, his way of always keeping his physical body fit. I enjoyed these things with him. These attributes are what I want in my husband and in our marriage.

"Then one day Dev asked me if I would go shopping with him to buy a sweatsuit. We went to a store and he went straight to the ladies' sizes and started looking through them. I was puzzled so I asked him who the suit was for. He told me that he wanted to buy it for me. I felt so special because he always treated me like a queen. He also took me on the job with him installing doors. We got very close talking and being together, and I felt really important when he thought enough of me to take me places like that with him. I loved him very much and I never wanted to do anything against his ideals or mine. He gave me the confidence I needed to succeed in the activities I was involved in. He never said one mean or discouraging word to me. I've always wanted to somehow pay him back for the way he treated me."

Dear Gayle. Her handwritten story was typical of all she was—so unselfish and so willing to serve others. She had a great capacity to love. I remembered how grateful I was for her attitude when Dev went on his mission. That was when they really got close. It all seemed to start on the night of his birthday party. Vicki had the family over to her place for Devro's nineteenth birthday. He was thinking about it that day. . . .

"Mom, do you think Vicki would care if I brought a date?"

"I don't think so. Why?"

"Well, the girls are always there with their husbands and I just like somebody to be with."

"I'm sure it will be just fine."

"Well, I don't want to go to the 'Y' to get any-one . . . what about Gayle? Do you think the girls like Gayle?"

"I don't think they know her well enough to like or dislike her. Bring her if you want to. Maybe we should get acquainted."

He hadn't heard my words; he went on as if he were talking to himself. "Yeah, I think I'll bring Gayle. I like being with her, and she lives close by."

And when he brought her that night, I was really impressed. I knew he had dated her, and he had talked to me about her, but this time I could see for myself. In the midst of that family situation, with the grandchildren jumping on Dev and with his sisters doting over him and so much talk among the men, Gayle didn't try to compete. She quietly kept herself busy with some of the younger children who were also feeling left out. She would read a story softly or play with the baby. Yet, when Dev needed her to help with the home movies, she was right there. That was another thing: home movies for anyone who isn't in them must really be a bore, but not for Gayle. She asked a few questions here and there, just enough to show us that she was really interested. I think the girls were prepared not to like her, but they couldn't help responding to her sweetness and her quiet way. She was the one girl Dev's cousin Kevin liked him to go with.

Kevin and Devro—cousins and best friends. They had been through a lot together, from Little League clear up to their missions. Kevin, six weeks older, received his mission call before Devro did, but the stake president gave special permission for them to go through the temple together.

That night we held the traditional family dinner, which was a custom with us whenever any of our family members went through the temple for the first time. What a party that was! Everybody was laughing and teasing.

"Boy, it's a good thing you two aren't going to the same mission, or the Church would be in rough hands."

"Yeah, we'd better put a couple of continents between these two."

"Well, Kevin is going to speak Spanish in the Buenos Aires North Mission. Maybe we can get them to let Devro speak Pig Latin."

The comments went on and on all evening, but the really amusing part came the next day when Devro got his call. He read it and laughed a full five minutes before he called Kevin.

"Hey, Kev, guess where I'm going on my mission?"

"Where are you going?"

"Buenos Aires!"

"Oh, sure. Now come on and tell me where you're going."

"I told you—Buenos Aires South Argentina."

"I don't believe you. I can't believe you—now, come on!"

But that was what it was—the same country, the same city, but different missions. It was a comforting thought, when they were both going so far away, that they would be in the same country and the same city some of the time.

Dev's farewell was held a few weeks later. I'll never forget that special day. Gayle attended the meeting but didn't let him take her.

"You'll need to be with your family today. I'll bring mine and come because I want to hear what you have to say. But I don't want you to worry about being with me when you have so many relatives and friends."

I guess a son's mission farewell is one of the high points of his mother's life. I was thrilled to see so many of Dev's friends and relatives gathered to share this occasion with him. Linda started things off with a tribute to Devro from his sisters, and various family members spoke and sang. Finally it was our missionary's turn. I'll never forget the testimony he bore that day.

"I'd like to tell my Heavenly Father right now that there's nothing in the world I wouldn't do for him. And I hope I can go out in the mission field and do the gospel justice, to seek out and find the people who need it. I would like to bear my testimony, brothers and sisters, that I know this church is true. Every day I gain a stronger testimony of the little things—a little more and a little more each day. It's so great. I really want to share it with other people, and I hope I can. I'm thankful for our prophet and that he guides this church today. I hope my Heavenly Father will bless me out in the mission field. When hard times come I can go to him. I have always gone to him, and there hasn't been once when he hasn't helped me out and strengthened me. There's just no way I can repay him, but I'm sure going to try.

"I thank you all for coming, and I say these things in the name of Jesus Christ. Amen."

Everyone came over to our house after the meeting for punch and cookies—everyone but Gayle. Dev had a wonderful time talking and reminiscing with old friends, but when all the guests had gone home, he quietly slipped away to find Gayle.

6

Dev had always said he would do anything for his Heavenly Father, and I wondered as I stood outside Gayle's hospital room how much he would be called upon to do now. He had always met each new trial of his life with his head high and a smile on his face. Dev was a boy you couldn't keep down for long, but this . . .

All his life he had worked to make himself worthy to be a good husband and father, to have children of his own, and to share his memories and goals with them. His children had been the first thing in his mind since his own childhood: he had always talked about his little girl, his little boy. In his mission all the elders teased him about the handmade baby clothes he bought to bring home. His answer to the popular Argentine talk of abortion was to have a tiny silver baby pacifier made into a necklace for him to wear. Dev was a family man. Surely, with his righteous goals Heavenly Father would bless him, would bless Gayle and Skyler.

Dev came out of Gayle's room, the ever-ready smile on his face. He kissed me.

"Mom, the doctor came in last night and was encouraged. He said she was doing better. He thinks she is going to make it. He says if she will just turn that corner—she's right at the crisis."

"Oh, bless you, dear, that's good news. And Skyler?"

"I don't know. He's holding his own." We walked down the hall toward the waiting room. "You know, Mom, this morning when I was having prayer with Skyler, I put my hands on his head and blessed him, and I just kind of saw a little vision in my mind. I could see Skyler, our firstborn, with his brothers and sisters—they were looking to him for guidance and he was there helping them along. I could see him so clearly. I don't know what Heavenly Father had in mind, but I've dedicated our lives to His service, to the gospel and His will. If Skyler can stay with us, I'll teach him to love his Heavenly Father and serve Him. He's my little son and I love him so; every time I talk to him he opens his eyes and looks at me as if he understands.''

I smiled and felt a warm glow of pride at being the mother of a boy like this. I could never do enough to be worthy of that honor. His voice was serious, but he was happy as he told me these things. There wasn't anything dramatic about what he said or the way he said it, just a feeling of deep faith, hope, and determination along with the gentle tenderness. I wanted to cry, but the tears could never have expressed all I was feeling.

"Dev, can I stay with Gayle while Jean gets some rest or while you go home and shower—or anything?''

"Jean went home last night for a while. We're all right. But maybe you can see Gayle this morning."

"All right.''

"As soon as the doctor comes out, I'll see."

A nurse called Devro to the telephone and he left me. I sat in the waiting room, thinking what a helpless feeling it was to want to ease the hurt, to kiss away the fears as I had done when Dev was little. But this whole thing had been so freakish. A nurse, a friend of Gayle's, had suggested that the toxemia should have been detected in the doctor's office when Gayle went for her check-ups. But she checked the records, and everything had been done. It was a freakish thing, as if it were according to plan, chosen and—

"Mom, you can see Gayle now."

I went into the intensive care room to stand beside her. She was so very ill. Her eyes were bandaged now, and the trachea breather made it impossible for her to talk. I put my cheek to hers and made my voice sound happy.

"Gayle, it's Mom, your Sealy Mom. I've been here most of the time, just in case there's anything I can do." I slipped my hand into hers, and she tightened her fingers on mine. I knew she understood. "Gayle, we're all praying for you. Talk to Heavenly Father, dear, talk in your mind. Ask him what he wants you to do. Just pray and pray. You will be blessed for all this that you are going through. Great blessings come from great sacrifices and pain. Heavenly Father always fulfills everything he promises."

A slight squeeze of my hand let me know she heard, and then Devro came back. I kissed them both good-bye.

"I'm going to the temple now. If I can't do any good here, perhaps I can there."

"Wait a minute, and I'll walk you to the elevator."

I waited outside Gayle's room again until Dev joined me. As we walked to the elevator together he talked, sounding more encouraged than he had before. She seemed so ill to me that I hurt all over just thinking about her. But I hadn't been with her every minute the way he had. He would have noticed even a slight change.

"Have you gotten any sleep?" I asked.

"Yes, Mom, Jean and I took turns last night. I went into that room down the hall for a couple of hours, but I can't sleep much. I'm afraid Jean won't wake me when Gayle wakes, and I want to be with her. She knows when I'm there, and I can't let her go through this alone."

"Bless you, Dev. Oh, by the way, in case I'm not there when you come home to shower, there's a new pair of pants and a sports shirt laid out by your bed downstairs. You don't mind, do you? It's all I could think of to do."

In answer he kissed me and held me tightly for a minute. He was so independent it was hard to do anything for him. He hadn't needed many clothes before—and he hadn't bought many because he and Gayle had been spending money on their house—but now, for wearing in the hospital, some nice casual things would be cooler. I had stopped by the store and prayed I would get the right size.

"I appreciate all you are doing, Mom. Thanks. I'll come home and change today if Gayle is all right."

I left then and again drove up to the temple and went through the session alone. In my heart I could not understand why Gayle's illness was lingering so long. The doctors had thought she would improve immediately when they took the baby. I prayed for peace and comfort and the knowledge to understand.

After the temple session I went home to fix dinner so Dev could eat if he came home. Then I cleaned the house. As I worked I prayed and prayed and prayed.

Dev made it home for a quick change. The clothes I had bought fit him well, and he smiled.

"I don't know how you do it, Mother. I'm hard to fit in pants. Gayle and I hunted and hunted for my last pair, and yet you walk in and pick some out without me and they fit perfectly."

"I have a secret code," I said, remembering how I had prayed in my heart. I didn't want little things to be discouraging for him too.

He ate quickly and then left to go back to the hospital. He reported no change: all the doctors would tell him was that Gayle's condition was stabilized.

Later, Milt and I went for a drive. I knew the girls had planned on visiting with Dev at the hospital—they and their husbands had taken dinner in for the members of Gayle's family and Dev—so we weren't in a big hurry. The doctor's words that morning had encouraged us. But when we finally reached the hospital, Linda met us by the elevator door in tears. She was crying so hard that she couldn't talk.

"Linda, what is it?" I grabbed her in my arms and she struggled for breath between sobs to try to tell us.

"G-Gayle . . . oh, Mother, she's dying."

"Linda—" I held her even tighter as I looked around, only to find others in tears as well. "Linda, is she gone?" I asked, almost afraid of what her answer would be.

"N-no, not yet, but she's so bad and Dev—"

"Where is Dev?"

"He's with her."

"She isn't gone yet. Let's pray, let's stand together and have a family prayer."

I put my arms around Linda and we went to the waiting room. Vicki came and joined us.

"What happened, Vicki?"

"We were all here. Dev said she had been about the same all day. He has been with Skyler a lot today because they were watching her so closely and wouldn't let him in as often. We put out the food we brought for Gayle's family, and Dev came to be with us; then suddenly a nurse appeared and told him to come quickly, that Gayle was very low. She told us all to come. Dev ran and gave Gayle a blessing right then, and I think she is calmed a little."

I left them and went down the hall. Dev was beside Gayle, leaning over her. "You can make it, Gayle. Hold on, I know you can make it. You're going to be all right."

I watched her responding to him, trying to breathe deeper. Then the doctor came in and asked Dev to leave. He came out into the hall to join me.

"Dev?"

He put his arm around me and we walked to where the others were waiting in little groups of two or three as they cried and tried to comfort each other. As we walked, Dev said, "I don't think she is going to die now. I think that part is past again."

"Can we have a family prayer, all of us together?"

"Yes, that would be good."

As we gathered together Dev spoke to all of us. His voice was firm and hopeful, his eyes full of tenderness but not tears.

"The doctor is with her now. He's trying some more things."

"Let's have our prayer," I said, putting my arms around Linda and Loni, whose face was red from crying.

As we stood there together, our heads bowed, Devro offered a prayer, thanking Heavenly Father for Gayle and asking his special attention and blessings for her. He

49

poured out his desires for her comfort, that she might rest and be healed. When he had finished I asked to be able to add my thoughts, and I prayed for those attending her that they might be guided to do what was best.

All of Gayle's immediate family and all of ours were there, as well as a few close friends. While we waited we talked and tried to comfort each other, and gradually the conversations became more positive and our fears began to subside.

"You know, Linda," I said, "only those who know Devro and Gayle can possibly know how hard this is for them. She doesn't want to leave him, I know that. He has such strong faith that our Father in heaven could heal her, but I know he isn't trying to hold on to her against our Father's will."

There was a fresh flow of tears from Linda. She loved Dev and Gayle so much, and she had always been so gentle and tenderhearted, that this was almost more than she could bear.

"Oh, Linda, I didn't mean to make you cry. I hope the crisis is past. But you know that if she does have to go, she will go unto the Lord with the satisfaction that she has already completed in her short life more than most people complete in years and years. Gayle has everything she needs for salvation. She has faced every problem squarely and has already conquered herself better than I have. She has married the man of her choice in the temple and she has a son. She is Dev's for all eternity—"

"All she ever wanted was Devro," said her mother, who was standing close enough to overhear what we said. She continued, "The first time she ever saw Devro, she came home and told me he was what she wanted. 'Do you think I could ever have him, Mother? Is there any way in this world I can ever live worthy to have him?' That's what she said to me."

"That's what she told me too, Jean. Dev or somebody better—she wouldn't settle for less. I sort of adopted her, Jean. I hope you haven't minded my sharing her with you."

"She always talked about you a lot. I know what you meant to her."

"We did talk a lot. I used to tell her that I didn't care what Dev did, whether they were romantic about each other or not—that she and I were friends and she was part mine."

That's the way it had always been for me. Since the first trip we took to Disneyland, she and Loni and I, when Dev was on his mission, I had known what a special person she was, what strong characteristics she had. Even though I didn't know then that she would someday be married to Dev, I knew he would search a long time before he ever found such qualities all in one person again.

I watched Dev across the hall as he comforted another family—first the father of a boy who had been in an accident and was not expected to live, and then the mother and the boy's sister—and I wondered how we could comfort Dev if Gayle didn't get well. But she would get well. Surely Heavenly Father knew how much Dev needed Gayle, knew what an inspiration and help she was to him and had always been through his mission.

I remembered back to that time just before he left. He had asked her to go with us, as a family, the night he was set apart. Before picking her up, he asked me what they could do afterward.

"I don't feel right being with her alone after I've been set apart for my mission. I thought of going to a show, but could you go with us?"

"I can't believe you want me. Yes, I can go, but what about just staying here? I could fix some snacks for you to eat in front of the fire."

"Will you be here?"

"Sure. I'll be fixing things for Sunday dinner and working right here in the kitchen."

So that was what they did. After Dev was set apart, he and Gayle came home with us to sit in front of the fire and eat snacks while they read their patriarchal blessings together.

When Dev was ready to take Gayle home, he came to find me. I was clearing up the kitchen.

"Mom, will you ride with me to take Gayle home?"

"Of course, but she only lives a few blocks away."

"I know, but I think it might be better if you were to come with us. The president didn't say I shouldn't be alone with a girl, but I know that is a rule and I would like to keep it."

"Fine. You can just call me a back seat driver." I laughed, but inside I was so very proud of him—a son who cared about details. I was sure the Lord would bless him.

We drove up to Gayle's house together and I waited in the car while he walked to the door with her. They stood on the front step a minute and then the door opened, sending a flood of light to silhouette the two of them as Dev held her hand. Then she went inside, the door closed, and Dev came back to the car.

"She's great, Mother. No tears, just a happy smile, and you know what she said? She said, 'Go get 'em, Dev!' She's really great!"

I didn't know Gayle very well then, but I wondered if she might be the one. Dev's sisters weren't too happy about his dating Gayle. She was still a little sister to them, and they thought she was too quiet and somewhat dull. But they didn't know her then; none of us really knew her. With her sterling qualities, she seemed too good to be true.

The next day was spent primarily in packing Devro's things. We made piles of everything that had to go into one suitcase: socks, white shirts, two suits with extra pants, and a thousand small items. We checked and re-checked; nothing could be left out, it all had to go. But we knew that not even a magician could fit all of that into the one suitcase Dev was to live out of for two whole years.

He sat there looking at it all while I hurried to finish last-minute details. I knew he was having a rough time; I had watched him through all the difficult days since his farewell as he had searched his heart. I knew the deep anxiety that comes to a young man leaving home for the first time, and I had seen the struggles Dev had experienced as he had wavered between his deep desire to serve his Father in heaven and his reluctance to part from his loves here at home. Now he sat looking out the window at his mountains. He looked at his dog, then got up and wandered around from room to room as if he wanted to drink in the sight of everything and soak it into his memory. He didn't talk much, and I didn't dare talk either. Finally, ignoring my urging to begin trying to fit everything into his suitcase, Dev went into his room, closed the door, and dialed a telephone number. He talked a long time, but when he came out he was smiling, and his whole attitude had changed.

That evening I said to my husband, "You know, Milt, that little Gayle just might be the girl Dev marries."

"Now, Shirl, don't start matchmaking. Dev is going on his mission and he hasn't time for girls."

"Right, and I wouldn't have it any other way. But I'm really not matchmaking. I just think—well, you know that Dev seldom gets down or discouraged, and if he ever does, nobody but me has ever been able to pull him out of it. But Gayle can. After talking to her, he's flying high again."

And there was another instance that made me think about Gayle. When we were standing in line at the mission home, Dev said to me, "Mom, while I'm away I want you to get acquainted with Gayle."

"Dev, do you think she might be the one?"

"I don't know. I do have a feeling that she will be here when I get home, and if she is . . . but we'll see. I want to marry whomever the Lord wants me to marry."

"Shirl . . ." Milt appeared in the doorway, jolting me back into the present. "Shirl, the doctors want to see Dev, Gayle's parents, and you and me for a minute."

We followed two doctors into a small room, where we all sat down. Then one of the doctors began to explain that they, the two of them with the advice of several others, had decided that Gayle's chances would be better if she could be taken to the LDS Hospital in Salt Lake City. There was some equipment there that wasn't available in Provo. They wanted to take her by ambulance as soon as possible. Skyler would be left where he was, in Utah Valley Hospital. We talked a while as the doctors explained all they could; then Dev made the decision that she should be moved. The doctors would take Gayle in the ambulance and Dev would follow in his car.

"This will mean I can't see Skyler as often," Dev said regretfully. "I wish the little guy could get better and his mother could get well enough to see him, just once, or hold him in her arms. Maybe this new equipment will help."

The boys blessed Gayle again, and as they rolled her to the exit the family began to disperse. At home, I waited for Dev's call; he had promised to let us know as soon as Gayle was settled. Milt was worn out with worrying. He felt so helpless in his desire to help Dev, and seeing what Gayle was going through was almost too much for him. He went to bed while I tried to fix my hair for the next day's speaking assignment. Finally, my hair finished, the house quiet, I reached for Gayle's journal again. There was an entry about Dev's mission and how she felt.

"Dev got his mission call to Argentina on March 8. The last day I was with him, before he left, we went to Scofield and stayed at my grandmother's and grandfather's house for the day. We ate lunch with them and sat and talked about 'the good old days.' Dev seemed to really enjoy my grandparents. I've always loved and respected my grandparents very much, and I felt that I would only introduce a very special young man to them, one who meant a lot to me. Dev didn't let me down. I've never regretted that special day. When Dev left on his mission, I was not sad and I did not cry. I was very happy, and I felt that I would see him again when he got home. I always had that peaceful reassurance within me."

What a help Gayle was to Devro on his mission! She

wrote faithfully and often, and her letters were full of encouragement. Dev wrote that he was lucky to have Gayle, because he watched other missionaries who received mushy letters from their girls and who became distracted from their labors. Gayle was especially careful. She had read an article containing advice on how to write to a missionary, and she was always careful to use that pattern.

Gayle and Loni started to get really close after Devro left. Gayle picked up Loni for karate; she said she was used to coming to the house anyway, and enjoyed picking up Loni. When she brought her home, sometimes we would talk or share lines from Dev's letters.

In one letter Dev wrote to Gayle after he entered the Language Training Mission, he reminded her that they hadn't made any promises or commitments, and that she was free to do whatever she wanted to do. He didn't want any room for hurts or disappointments.

When she read that letter, she got the point and fired one back to him. "Listen, I said I would support you on your mission. That means I will write to you as often as I can, whether you write or not, until I'm married." So the letter-writing continued while Devro prepared to leave for Argentina and Gayle prepared to graduate from high school and to go to Weber State College.

7

All my life I had heard of the wonderful blessings that come to the family of a missionary and to the missionary himself when he goes on his mission. I had never experienced these blessings before, since we had had only girls until Devro. But the blessings that came with Devro's mission I felt and knew and witnessed in my life and in my mind, though I can't fully explain them. I can tell how we watched for the mail and looked forward to running to the mailbox at the end of the lane. When a letter came from Dev, Loni and I would curl up on the couch with it and drink in the whole thing; then I would call the girls and share it with them, and if there was a message for Gayle, I would call her. We had a new closeness, a togetherness in all we did. And if Devro needed more money, somehow we had it, every time.

The Language Training Mission program was very hard for Devro. He had never studied a language before. When he took the language test, prior to receiving his call, he said, "Mother, I did the very best I could, and even though I haven't had any classes in any language, I don't think my test will hold me up if I'm called to a foreign mission."

We knelt together that day when all the papers were sent in, and prayed that those who selected Dev's mission would be guided as to where he should go, where his particular talents were needed. Dev hadn't given any preference or any hint of anything that might influence a decision. He hadn't even said that his grandmother came from Norway because he thought that might influence those who decided. He wanted to go where the Lord wanted him to be. When the call came for Argentina, there was no doubt in his mind that this was where he was meant to go. So even when learning the language was so hard, it seemed almost impossible, even when others could grasp it and he couldn't, he knew somehow he would be able to say what he needed to say in the service of his Father in heaven. There were other problems, too. I caught one paragraph as I turned the pages of his old letters: "By the way, I got a new companion and he is so straight. He doesn't like sports and hates to run. He won't laugh or joke or really express himself, but I guess the Lord has a purpose in putting us together. Maybe he's good for me."

And Gayle wrote such wonderful, encouraging things, like this: "At 5:45 A.M. I climbed out of my bed and said a very special prayer for you. It made me tingle all over, and I've felt so good all day that I just know everything is going right for you. Please don't worry about writing to me. As long as I know that my letters are welcome, I am content."

Dev wrote to her: "Most of the missionaries get letters from their girl friends that are so mushy, and all it does is make them wonder why they are out here. Not you! You support me and make me happy to serve.

"Gayle, don't forget that you can do anything you want to do. Some people are bound because they don't listen to the counsel of the Lord, but not you . . . so shoot for the stars and get what you want out of life. Be happy helping other people and know that you can accomplish anything you want to. Remember, whether you think you can or can't . . . you are right."

There was another one from Gayle—a look into her heart: "Dev, I've had so many prayers answered that there is no doubt in my mind that we have a Father who is listening. I love him so much that I can kneel beside my bed and tell him what is on my mind, just as though he were sitting next to me."

Throughout her memory books, everywhere I looked there was evidence of Gayle's deep testimony and her love for her Heavenly Father. How close she had always stayed! Yes, Heavenly Father would bless her and her baby; I was sure of it. I didn't know just how, but he was mindful of this girl who wanted only to be obedient. And Devro was the same; there was one letter that told of another experience he had had before leaving the Language Training School for Argentina:

"In the temple today I had an experience that is worth all of the struggle or any tough task in my whole life. My companion and I were asked to be witnesses for a special sealing. We went into the room and while we waited the temple worker explained that a little six-year-old boy's parents had been killed and his aunt and uncle, whom he hardly knew, were having him sealed to his parents. The spirit in the room was so strong as the little boy entered, holding the hand of a sweet lady temple worker. The little boy had the brightest, sweetest smile, a glow of joy like I've never seen before. Being the big baby that I am, the tears rolled down my face. I was so happy for him. As they knelt at the altar and he was sealed to his parents for time and all eternity, the little boy glowed forth even brighter with the biggest smile I have ever seen. Quite a young man was he. That experience was so great and wonderful I can't even relate it properly. I have so many great things happening to me."

Events rolled on. Dev was facing one thing after another, and Gayle was getting ready for graduation. Dev wrote: "I wish I could be there to see you walk down the aisle and watch the look on your parents' faces—that look of pride—but all I can give you for graduation is the love of my heart and a thank you for all of your letters and everything you have done to support me."

A seminary teacher had once challenged Gayle to write a letter to her future husband. She had put the letter—a letter Dev had never read—in her personal memory book, and my eyes scanned it now:

"TO MY FUTURE HUSBAND:

"Today I have moved away from home into an apartment which I hope to make my home. It is so hard for me to completely leave my family because I love them so much. Whenever I'm away from them I have a lonely, empty feeling inside that seems to take over all my thoughts. The fun things we did together keep coming back to my mind, and so I sit and wish I were back with them again. I keep telling myself that I must break away and lead a life of my own until I have found the one with whom I will start a family of my own. I know you are out there somewhere, but I am not quite ready to find you.

"I want to be the type of wife that my Heavenly Father would have me be for you. I want to be your friend in every way and I want to be your eternal partner. I want to be a pure woman who will bring precious spirits into this world. I want to be a handmaiden of the Lord in teaching these special spirits. I want us to become a family who have great love for each other, a love that is far better than any other. Together we will grow toward our celestial goal, and together we will reach it. I want to support you in your priesthood callings because I know you are a special man who has a unique purpose on this earth.

"I am so thankful that I have learned in my youth that the power of creation is sacred, and I am so thankful that I have lived up to the standards of the Lord. A kiss to me is very sacred, and as I date now I refuse to give any of them away. I know that when I am ready to find you, you will be the one to get my kisses. Even though I will find you, my kisses will still be sacred and very few until we are sealed under an everlasting covenant. After we are married, we will always respect each other and never use or mistreat each other. We have been given a very sacred power, which we will use the way the Lord has commanded us. I will love bearing our children, and their number is not limited in my eyes. I want to have as many as the Lord will give us.

"Right now I have feelings that I know who you are, but I must still prepare myself as though I have not yet found you. To me you are the image of a strong, healthy man who cares enough about his body to keep it in good shape. You are a great man who stays on a spiritual track. You are a man who can smile and laugh and have fun. You are very strong, but you are also very humble, meek, and quiet. You love our Father and want to be forever in His service. You will do anything for Him. I know we will become the great unit that a man and woman should become. I know I will be the right person for you when I have reached the goals I have set for myself. I will always be reaching because what I want to give to you is everlasting."

I closed the book thinking, *Gayle, my Gayle, as much a part of my life as Dev even though I haven't known you as long. Oh, Father in heaven, bless her, please bless her. She has lived such a good life and has such beautiful goals.*

The telephone rang and I ran to answer it.

"Mother?"

"Yes, Dev. Is Gayle all right?"

"Yes, she's stabilized again. We had a real scary trip."

"Scary how?"

"I was driving behind the ambulance and it had a blowout."

"A blowout? I thought it was a new one."

"It was a brand new one, but it had a blowout. But you know, it just barely wiggled. I couldn't believe it. By all the laws it should have been thrown off the road. And then the new one we called got there in five minutes. One of the doctors said he couldn't believe it and thought we must have someone special upstairs looking over us."

"It could have caused a lot of trouble with the machines if they hadn't gotten another right away. They were really sweating it! But it's all right now. She's settled and they give her a fifty-fifty chance. If only she will turn that corner and show some healing."

"Don't hesitate to call if you need anything, Devro."

"I won't, Mom. I guess my phone bill is going to be terrible, and my business is just hanging, but I'm not going to leave her, no matter what."

"Don't worry about anything here."

"I called about Skyler and he's still holding his own. I hate to be so far away from him. If Gayle is all right, I'll come down in the morning."

"Vicki said she would go, too. I have to speak in the morning up at Aspen Grove, but I'll go down to the hospital in the afternoon."

"Thanks, Mom, and thank Vicki. I think I told her, but—"

"I'll let her know. I hope you can get some rest."

"There's a couch here and the nurse gave us some blankets and pillows. This waiting room is right next to the intensive care lab where Gayle is, so I can go in whenever they will let me."

"You're not alone, then?"

"No, Jean and Gayle's father, Stan, are here. I'm sure glad Stan got here. We're going to have prayer and then bed down. Gayle is resting. They gave her something to help her sleep."

"I'll try and sleep too, then. Remember—call."

There was a click and I put the phone down. Passing through the kitchen on my way to bed, I stopped to get a drink. I drank half a glass of water and poured the rest on a dry plant. *Gayle's plants must be getting dry*, I thought. *Dev hasn't been home. I must remember to get a key made from his so I can water her plants tomorrow.*

*T*he early morning drive up Provo canyon to Aspen Grove was inspirational beyond belief, in view of the mental and spiritual shock my soul was trying to grasp and absorb. The sharpness of nature's beauty around me touched me with reality and brought a sense of security, taking me out of the realm of mental anguish. Fasting had sharpened my senses, and I seemed to view the limitation of life on this earth in comparison with what was before and what would come after. I fought against thinking about Gayle and Skyler, yet nothing else was possible, and inwardly I still cried out for knowledge and understanding of my role in this plan of our Father's.

I knew we were all feeling more than we had the mental capacity to understand. I had called Linda and Vicki before I left, and there was that hurt in both their voices. Everyone wanted to do something, to help, to give—and yet, more than ever, I was aware that all past and future events were in the hands of a greater power than any of us possessed.

I arrived at the grove to face a group of eager, beautiful young ladies, and to speak to them about the beauty of the gospel and about the power of purity. I was uplifted by the Spirit, which seemed to talk through me, and as I drove down the canyon I decided to visit the hospital before going home.

Washed and scrubbed, I stood beside Skyler's little waterbed. I put one finger into his hand and felt his fingers tighten as he opened his sky blue eyes and looked at me. How strong his little spirit was, even though his body was weak! I felt hallowed just being in the presence of a spirit so recently come from our Father.

"Little baby Skyler," I whispered softly as I rubbed his little feet. I knew no one else could hear me because of the sounds of the machinery that recorded his progress. "How special you are, how wise—if only you could talk, you could answer all my confusions. Do you know, little grandson, you look just like your daddy? And that means your mother too, because I think your mother and father look alike." I hummed a little song and felt better for having visited.

Later that afternoon I drove up to the hospital in Salt Lake City to take Dev some food and fresh clothes. He could shower at his sister Judy's house. Having Judy and her husband, Neal, close to the LDS Hospital was a comfort to Dev—help at his fingertips, if he needed it. Gayle's mother had gone to freshen up when I got there, so I was allowed to sit beside Gayle's bed and feel of her spirit as I had felt Skyler's. How much could she tell me if she could really talk? There seemed to be a special bond between Gayle, her son, and that world beyond.

Outside her room I was aware of the suffering of other people around us. And I knew that we, as a family, because of the gospel, were more equipped to bear what we were experiencing than were many others. Talking to different people who had come to wait, to cry, and to pray, I found that Devro had already been an influence and comfort to many. Listening to the heartaches of others made the time rush past, and soon Devro was back. He was smiling, smelling like fresh soap, and he rushed past me with a quick greeting as he went in to see Gayle.

The telephone in the corner of the waiting room rang, and I went to answer it. It was Linda.

"Mother, what about Gayle?"

"No change. Just the same."

"Both meetings in our ward today were practically dedicated to Gayle and Dev. In Sunday School the bishopric asked for those who hadn't yet heard about our ward fast to start fasting, and Brother Ron cried when he told of the great need. There is such love here. The fast meeting was the same; everyone was so concerned and so many people have been affected by Gayle's and Dev's lives."

"Oh, Linda, I can't believe how many people have gone out of their way to show their love and concern."

"I can't get it off my mind either, Mother. You know the pain I've been having in my knees? The doctor said it was arthritis from worry. That made me mad at myself. I've got to get hold of my feelings . . . if only there was some way I could help."

"I know, Linda, but you have to go on with your life and not let your feelings of concern make you ill. You have children and a husband depending on you, and we have to go on. We never know who will be next."

"I guess that's why we feel so sympathetic. This could happen to any of us."

There were other calls—cousins to say they were getting blood donors, people we hadn't heard from in years—and then Jean came back and I went home. The house was quiet again. I needed to get some rest, but I was restless. My mind was still on Gayle and Dev and that sweet love, so young and perfect, between them.

How the letters had passed back and forth! I couldn't believe how many letters Gayle had written to Dev; she had sent quite a few tapes too. And she had mounted all the letters Dev had written to her in a special book. I opened her memory book again and came across a picture of her in her karate outfit. She had earned a brown belt in karate. She was always working on something.

Gayle had decided on a degree in interior design at college. While she went to school, as if that wasn't enough, she also got a job decorating for one of the stores, which gave her practical experience in her field. She was always thrifty with her money, and with what she saved from her job, she was able to take flying lessons on the side. She wasn't sure Dev would approve. One letter said:

"Dev, I hope you aren't too disappointed in me for taking flying lessons. Even if I am a girl, I need to learn all I possibly can. And when you come home, I know you will get a chance to start flying too, if you want to. And you can pass me up because I'm not taking lessons very often. But it is a blast, and I know you'll dig it. Did I hear a note of jealousy in your last letter? Don't worry about the guy who got me started. He is a returned missionary and he is super nice, but too mature for me and his bald head doesn't appeal to me romantically—not at my age. He's just a nice friend."

Dev was having some problems at this time. His letters weren't getting through for quite a while, and we were anxious. I wrote him twice a week because I wasn't sure which letters, if any, he would receive. Then we finally heard that he was all right, but a hundred people had been gunned down about fourteen blocks from where he was.

I turned a page in Gayle's journal, and there was an entry she had made close to the end of Dev's mission: "I've written to Devro twenty-one months of his mission and I've enjoyed every minute. He wrote to me a lot at first, sending tapes every once in a while during the first year. He soon slowed down, and I knew that he was dedicating his whole effort to his mission. I feel very proud to be associated with that great man. He has written me, I'm sure, his last letter, saying that he really loves me but that he feels uneasy about what might happen when he comes home. I don't blame him for feeling that way, because I feel the same way. I don't want to ever be an obligation to anyone. If Dev is to take me out when he gets home, he will have to want to take me out, not take me out because he feels he has to. It will be interesting to see how things turn out."

Gayle had done her work. She and Dev agreed to stop writing, and she began to think more seriously of other boys. Yet she didn't give up or lose track of Dev. Whenever she came home for a weekend, she called me or ran in to listen to a tape. She did this quietly because she cared, but Dev didn't ever know. I didn't tell him, and she wasn't writing to him then. During this time Gayle made another entry in her journal:

"I've written to another missionary his full two years. The relationship was only friends and I thought it would always stay that way, but two months ago he returned home and things changed. I started to really love him but not enough to marry him. I told him that I needed more time to get to know him. We did many things together, but every time we saw each other, we had stupid disagreements. He didn't treat me as I believe a guy should treat a girl. On Christmas Day we had our usual disagreement and after a long moment of silence, he casually said, 'Maybe we should forget the whole thing.' I knew right then that it would never work. I took what he said seriously, and agreed with him. We said our good-byes, but he didn't think they were for real. He called the next morning and said he had thought things over and felt he must talk to me again. We drove up the canyon together and talked, but I felt even stronger about my decision and I knew, for sure, that he wasn't the one I wanted to marry. It has now been a week since that time, and I'm hoping I will not have to see him again. I will always have a great love for him, and because of our relationship, I have learned a lot that will help my future relationship with my husband."

Meanwhile Dev, in the mission field, was facing some rough challenges himself. He had some really frightening bouts with sickness and accidents, but the blessings of the priesthood and medicine brought him through all right. His reports of the missionary work were glowing and full of wonder. About eight months before he was to come home, we received a tape:

"The last zone conference, the president called me in for my interview and after a few minutes he gave me a big hug and said: 'Elder Sealy, what would you think about being a branch president?' I said, 'Well, I'll do whatever the Lord wants me to do.' That's all he said then except that he wanted me to think about it. I didn't really think I would be called. But this Sunday the call came and the president came down here to be with me and let his counselors take over at a conference. He is so wonderful. And now I feel good about the call, and I'm not too worried, because when the members were told, they seemed happy. I think I have a lot of respect here, at least for now. I'm surprised at how the Lord works to prepare us for the callings that he gives us.

"I really had a fight with myself because I knew there might be an opening for a branch president here and I didn't want it, really I didn't. It's a good thing I always want to do what the Lord calls me to do. I've prayed and I've prayed so much, but it came and I'm happy, happier than ever. I'm so busy I don't know which way is up, but with time and the help of the Lord, things will be straightened out and I'll still be able to complete my missionary goals. I know I will."

Gayle came home that weekend and called me. When I told her I had a tape she slipped up, even though the house was full of people, went into Dev's room, turned on the tape, and listened. She always seemed to love the quiet moments she had alone in Dev's room with his voice on a tape. When she opened the door and came out, I could tell she had been crying, but her tears were tears of pride.

Even though Gayle was away at school it was obvious that her heart was still at home. In her file was a letter she had written to her mother that let me know how strong her ties at home were, and how they also fit into her program of always searching for ways to improve herself. She wrote home:

"Mom, I feel I must write this letter because I need your help. Lately I've been searching into my life for all the sins I've committed that I need to repent of. The only things I can think of are things that I question how to repent of. I'm sure you remember when I was smaller I had the problem of getting into your drawers. I don't know what was wrong with me because you had taught me well. But I don't do that any more so I guess I've outgrown it. Maybe that will take care of my repentance on that, but what I need your help with right now is, how can I repent of taking something from a store without paying for it?

"Mom, I was about ten when this happened and can you believe that it has been bothering me for eight years? It seems so small, but it has been eating at me for so long that it is really big. I've thought about going to the store and paying for it, but I don't know how I could do it; the same people aren't there now. This really seems dumb, but it isn't because I need your help to know how to repent of this. I was sent to you as your earthly daughter, and you are here to teach and guide me back to our Father in heaven. I need to take advantage of your purpose. I want to gain eternal life so badly. I would do anything that is asked of me to get it.

"Mom, it won't be long before I will have the opportunity to teach a daughter of my own. How could I ever do this if I haven't done all the things I should do before guiding her back to Heavenly Father?"

"Mom, I know there are still little things that hold my spiritual growth back and I'm sure you recognize them. I surely would appreciate it if you would let me know about them. I need a lot of help.

"Thanks for all you and Dad do for me. You are the greatest parents."

I looked further, and there, put together, were two letters. I knew Gayle's mother must have given her some help as to how to repent of the small things that were bothering her, for these two letters were filed next to the one she had sent to her mother.
"Dear Sir:

"I am writing this letter because of a foolish mistake I made when I was about 10 years old that has caused me a lot of pain.

"One day, while walking through your store, I took a bracelet that was worth about five dollars. I've hated myself for years because of this one act.

"I don't know quite how to ask for your forgiveness and pay for what I took, but I hope this is a way of doing it. I know the owners of the store have changed, so could you please give this letter to the person who had to pay for the loss?

"I will gladly do whatever I can to make up for your loss and free my conscience. Please reply soon so I will know what you would like me to do to make up for what I have done. Sincerely, Gayle Burch."

And the answer came shortly:

"Dear Miss Burch:

"After having given your letter to past and present management, they have asked that I write to you. We are very much pleased that in these troubled times when personal honesty seems to be a thing of the past, you would want to clear up such a matter. We compliment you. Prior management as well as present management want you to feel free from this matter and require nothing further of you. Again, our compliments to you."

The letter was signed by the local store manager, and as I put both letters back in the place where I had found them, I thought how really special this daughter-in-law of mine was. In all the talks we had had, she had never told me about this. Most people would have shown the letter because of the praise she received, but not Gayle. Gayle knew how to repent of even the smallest wrong. She could never flaunt her goodness.

Once more I closed Gayle's memory book. I began to get ready for bed while I waited for Dev to call before he settled down for the night. Would he report that she was better? I was praying she would be better this time. I had never known a girl who was so diligent in righteousness. Surely she had earned a blessing. Yet, I knew she would want to do whatever her Heavenly Father wanted her to do. As much as she loved her husband and son, as much as she wanted to stay and be with them, I knew that if Heavenly Father called her, she would respond. Our Father's call was the only one that would ever ring above the call of her husband. Yet, wasn't that why she had always responded to her husband so readily—because he also loved and responded to the wishes of our Father in heaven?

*D*ev's report was that Gayle was having a bad time again. Skyler wasn't doing very well either. It was strange the way they seemed to respond to each other even though they were miles apart. They had both developed some kind of pneumonia in their lungs.

"Oh, Dev," I cried.

"I've been with her all morning as much as they would let me."

"Shall I bring you some clothes and food?"

"No. Jean is here now and I think I'll come home and shower."

"I'll have some food ready for you."

"I don't know about eating. Everything kind of sticks in my throat."

"Well, it will be ready in case you feel like eating. I love you, Dev."

"Thanks, Mom, I love you too."

He hung up. He had sounded so discouraged, more than ever before since they had taken her to the Salt Lake hospital. Gayle was in pain and heavily sedated now, and that left him feeling alone. As long as she could squeeze his hand and nod her head to his questions, he had held up pretty well, but now . . . well, he was holding tight to his faith.

Dev came home a little after that. He showered and changed clothes and then came to sit beside the table, look at his food, and talk.

"I'm going to the temple, Mother. Maybe I can think more clearly there. I'm getting so I can't think anymore."

"I know, Dev." I said the words, but they were crazy: I didn't *know*. All I could do to empathize was to take what I was feeling and multiply it by a thousand. But I did care. "Dev, do you want me to go to the hospital to be with Gayle?"

"That would be nice, Mother. Jean is getting so tired."

I drove up to the hospital thinking about Devro and how discouraged and down he was. I hoped the temple calmness might give him courage. As I drove the tears came to my eyes. I blinked them back. I couldn't cry yet; Gayle needed strength and courage, not tears. Someday soon now she would be feeling better, and then I would sit down and really cry, I thought.

Off the freeway into Salt Lake traffic, I stopped at a red light thinking, *Oh, Father, if you need someone, please take me instead of Gayle. Can't I do what you might need? Or is this just a testing period for us all?* The light changed and I started forward just as a car on my left ran the red light. Automatically I put on my brake, and he barely missed me. How easily I could have been hit, but evidently the time wasn't right. I had two other close calls on the way up to the hospital, and by then I knew that I had extra protection and that no matter what I wanted to do for Gayle, I couldn't bargain with my life. I was being told no.

At the hospital I sat by Gayle while Jean went down for dinner. She was not responding to anything. A cold feeling ran over my body and I found it hard to swallow. Now I could see why Devro had been so discouraged: he couldn't stand to see her there, suffering so. The telephone rang and I answered it. It was Devro.

"Mom, is there any change?"

"Not any they have told me about, and the doctors' reports aren't good."

"Oh, Mom, I don't know what to do anymore."

"Maybe you need some sleep. Why don't you sleep a little while?"

"I can't. I couldn't even relax my mind in the temple. I don't know what is expected anymore."

"Why don't you come up here?"

"I will. I'll be up in a while."

I hung up the phone. I had never heard that catch of discouragement in Dev's voice before. He had always faced everything and had known what to do—Dev, who always bounced back so quickly. What could I do to help him?

The nurse called me: Gayle was rousing for the first time in hours. I went to her bedside, put my hand in hers, and felt a pressure.

"I'm here, Gayle. It's Shirl. I love you, Gayle."

I watched her lips form the words, "I love you." There was a good feeling, even though she was so terribly ill. Her lips were moving again, but I couldn't make out the words.

"Gayle, I can't understand. Say it again." I watched while she carefully mouthed words, and finally I dared ask, "Gayle, have you been praying?"

She nodded.

"Do you know what Heavenly Father wants?"

She nodded again.

"Can you stay with us and get better?"

She shook her head and moved her lips again, and I thought I saw her form the word "die."

"Gayle, do you want to die?"

She waited a minute and then nodded. But she formed the word "Dev."

"You want Dev?"

She shook her head.

I tried again: "Are you worried about Dev?"

She nodded.

"Don't worry about him, honey. Whatever is best for you he will understand. Do you want to go back to Heavenly Father?"

She nodded slowly. I sat down in a chair beside her and wondered if she knew what she was saying or if she was somewhere in a fog of incomprehension. Yet she seemed to know what she was saying, and I had a feeling she knew more than she could say, and was trying to communicate it to me. Her mother came in and we both went through the process again. Then the nurses asked us to leave for a while and we went out into the waiting room.

"I wonder if she knows how ill she is?"

Jean shook her head as she said, "I don't know. She seems to know everything."

"But Gayle has always been a fighter. She has conquered everything she has ever tried."

"I know. Now she seems to want to give up." Jean wasn't crying as she said it. She had watched her daughter suffer and struggle too long to oppose anything. I knew we both wanted only what was best for Gayle.

"But Jean, what will Dev do without her?"

"I don't know—or if she can be happy anywhere without Dev. He put the smile on her face. He's made her so happy."

"She did everything with him. They went shopping for baby clothes just before she got sick. Gayle told me they had planned on buying something every week for the baby, but they got a little behind on their shopping, so just before her illness they went downtown and bought several things to catch up. And she has made such darling things. If Gayle dies, do you think the baby will die too?"

"I don't know. It's strange the way they seem to do everything together, almost as if they are still attached."

"Jean, what if I call the bishop—but I guess we had better wait for Dev."

"We won't have to wait long—here he comes."

I looked up and there was Dev, his long stride bringing him toward us. He was smiling and didn't look at all as he had sounded on the phone a few minutes before. He passed us and went to put on a gown, wash up, and go in to Gayle. We waited. He was with her a few minutes and then came out.

"She's conscious. She can squeeze my hand again." He sat down by us. "Did she try to say anything to you?"

I told him the experience we had had, and when the nurse would let him back in, he went to talk to her. He came back a few minutes later with tears in his eyes.

"She does. She wants to die." The tears spilled over and his chin quivered.

I put my hand on his arm and asked, "Dev, would you like to have the bishop come up and help give her another blessing? Maybe she doesn't know what she's saying."

"I do need someone with me. And what about Dad?"

"He's on his way. He called a little while ago; he's coming here from work."

"Call the bishop, Mom, and call Judy and Neal." Dev was a "family-ized" boy, and though he didn't want to work a hardship on anyone's schedule, he wanted his family around him now.

I couldn't reach the bishop, so I called another friend of the family, a very spiritual man. He promised to come right up.

Dev waited beside Gayle. She was so ill that she was incoherent part of the time, and the other times we weren't sure. As soon as our friend arrived we all gathered around Gayle's bed and Dev gave her a blessing, a sweet blessing as only a boy with his wholehearted devotion could give.

He dedicated Gayle to her Heavenly Father and asked him to do what was best for her. As he finished the prayer, Gayle lifted her weak arms, as if she knew everything that was going on, and with Dev's help got them clear up around his neck. He held her until her arms fell and we thought she had gone, but she was only resting in a half-conscious state. Then we went out into the waiting room and sat, thinking she was dying. The magic of that beautiful scene and the strength of Dev's attitude made it an inspirational moment. I suggested that maybe Judy and Neal would like to go home, since Judy was expecting her fourth baby, and the waiting facilities were uncomfortable. Neal consulted with her and then said, "We'd like to stay, if it's all right. There's a beautiful spirit here with Gayle, and we'd like to be part of it." We relaxed back into our chairs. Our friend put his arm around Dev.

"Dev, you're a good man. I don't know if I would have

the courage to do what you have just done. Your obedience is something wonderful to see.''

The hospital was quiet now, except for the sound of the machinery working. The lights were out except where we sat. We waited, making ourselves as comfortable as we could on the chairs, the straight-back couch, or the floor. There were books there beside us, but I could only think of Dev and Gayle—and Skyler. What would happen to Skyler, if Gayle died? We had two families who would love to raise that sweet little boy. I thought of him, and knew Vicki had visited him that day and Dev had seen him too. It was so important that he knew he was loved. Love was important to us all right now. Dev had always had a lot of love and a lot of confidence, but it had been Gayle's love for him and his for her that had given him this kind of courage. And to think there had been a time when he didn't even want to see her. I thought back to that time in both their lives, those weeks just before he came home from his mission. Gayle had written in her journal:

"The last time I wrote in my journal was just as I broke up with a missionary. Two days after I said good-bye to my missionary, whom I had decided never to marry, I met another man whom I had only known from a distance before. I dated him for almost four months. He was twenty-four, the same age as my sister's husband was when she was my age. I don't think he liked me very much at first, but as time went on he began to fall in love. I grew to love him too, but as time went on, I knew Devro would be coming home soon. I still had a lot of strong feelings for Devro. I knew I wasn't ready to get married until I saw Devro again. I knew my friend was getting anxious to get married, but he agreed with me that all of my feelings had to be sure. I had to see whom I loved the most, him or Devro."

At that same time Devro wrote home from the mission field: "Hope you received my letter about my staying an extra two weeks. Mom, I don't want any GIRLS at the airport when you come to pick me up, OK? That is, not any but the family—no girl friends, ex-girl friends, etc. I would appreciate it if you would take care of this."

I didn't have to tell Gayle. She had already decided that if Dev wanted to see her, he would have to come to Weber College to find her. But she came home to hear the last tape Dev sent before he left the mission and the branch. It was a heartrending tape, full of love and service, from an overtired boy completing his goals and trying to leave his branch with everything complete. He was tired. I could hear it in his voice as the tape drawled on, as if he were talking with his eyes shut. And yet there was such depth and love in his voice, such humility and heartache. Just before he signed off he said:

"There's been a lot of illness in the branch and we've been blessing a lot of people. Everywhere I go the people say, 'Presidente, you need some sleep,' and I tell them I'll get some when I get home. . . . See you at the airport. 'Bye for now."

I cried and cried when I got that tape. I was so proud to be his mother and so glad he was coming home where he could get medical attention from our own doctors and where I could give him his vitamins and good food suited to his system. I didn't tell Gayle about that tape, but somehow she sensed it was time and called me to ask. I told her about it then, and she hurried up to listen to the tape before going back to school. And she cried and cried too. As the tape finished, she remarked, "Nobody will ever know what he has been through, how hard he has worked, and how much he has accomplished. He's a great man."

My thoughts reverted back to the hospital and those around me as Dev came out of Gayle's room. I looked up inquiringly but didn't want to wake the others if they were sleeping. Dev saw my look and stepped closer.

"Mom, she's still unconscious, but her signs look better. Maybe she isn't going to die."

"You just go on," said our friend, rousing. Then I

76

knew he hadn't been asleep at all, but just thinking. He got up and put his arm around Dev again. "You go on living by the Spirit, Dev. Heavenly Father won't allow you to make any mistakes."

Dev grasped his hand.

"Dev, I'm going to leave now," he said, "but I'll come by in the morning, and if there is any change or you need anything before then, just call."

Dev walked to the elevator. Milt roused and offered to go home to take care of things there while I stayed with Devro. We said our good-byes; then Dev and I talked a little before settling down to wait for morning or for a change in Gayle.

I tried to sleep, but my mind went on with Devro's and Gayle's story. I would never forget the day he came home from his mission or the moving events of the days and weeks that followed.

10

Devro was coming home! After two years, plus a two-week extension, our missionary was coming home. What a magic moment it was when we saw him emerging from the airplane! He was so thin, so pale, but he wore a magnificent smile and glowed with the spirit of one who had been serving the Lord with all his heart, might, mind, and strength. And even though the hour was late, the family—brothers, sisters, nieces and nephews, in-laws, cousins, uncles and aunts—as well as bishops and friends, turned out to line up and greet him. He couldn't believe that reception!

My contribution to the celebration had been to fix all Dev's favorite foods for Sunday dinner, but he couldn't eat much; the food made him ill. And he had a lump on his leg that frightened me, though I didn't say anything about it to him. I had made a doctor's appointment for him for the next day, so we would wait until then to worry.

As I told Dev good night after an exhausting day of greeting and talking and settling in, he said, "I don't think I'll go to see Gayle."

"All right."

"I think it will be best if I don't. I've got a lot to do. I want to finish college and start a business. Mom, I'm fascinated with making money and I know I can. It's not that I care so much about money, I just want to make a lot of it so I won't have to worry financially while I get my schooling and go on serving the Lord. I would like to be worthy to serve another mission some time—not as a single missionary, but with my wife, when I find her—and that will take financial independence. I just think I won't see Gayle. I don't want to hurt anybody."

"All right, but I'm sure she doesn't expect anything."

There wasn't any more talk, but that night, while I was trying to settle my excitement and get some sleep, the lump in Dev's leg worried me. I knew enough about medicine to worry about cancer; the thought haunted me all night as I imagined what the doctor might say the next day.

Then, toward morning, after I had prayed most of the night, I realized that this was what Satan wanted me to think. I was forgetting the Lord's plan, forgetting that Devro had always been in his hands. I reproached myself for being so foolish, and mentally told Satan to get out of my life, as Devro had always done when he was young.

The next morning we prayed for wisdom on the part of the doctor and those who would examine Dev that day, and we left for town. In the car Dev said, "Maybe it wouldn't hurt to go see Gayle. I do care about her and want her to be happy."

"Why not? You're good friends and you've been through a lot together."

"Yes, I guess that wouldn't hurt. Do you think she's home?"

"I don't know. She usually comes home only on weekends."

"Maybe I'll call her when we get back."

"Are you afraid of meeting her, of what she might be feeling?"

"No, I'm more afraid of myself. I might like her, and I won't have time for girls for a long time."

We didn't talk any more; we had to go to the lab for tests and then to the store to get Dev a suit and some casual pants. He had left everything he owned, except the clothes he wore, with the people of his branch whom he loved so much. When we were finished shopping it still wasn't time for his doctor's appointment, so we went to look for a watch for him. The wristwatch he had had for his mission was no longer working. He thought a digital watch would be nice, and he had a little money in his savings account.

We didn't find the watch Dev wanted for the price he wanted to pay, but as we stood there waiting by the counter he looked at the diamonds. We laughed about how soon he might need one, and then we heard the owner say that diamonds were taking a big jump in price. He had just received notice that the price would go up twenty percent the next day. Dev was interested, and he decided that a diamond would be a good investment. Suddenly, before either of us knew it, he was making a down payment on a diamond without a setting.

As we drove to the doctor's office he was suddenly embarrassed.

"Don't tell anyone."

"I wouldn't think of it."

"It's just a good investment."

"That's right, just a good investment."

"And then, you never know how soon I may need one."

We arrived at the doctor's office and had to wait only for a few minutes. When the doctor looked at the lump on Dev's leg, I could see he was worried, too. He asked Dev a lot of questions, and then, as an afterthought, said, "Let's look at your toes. Have you had any infection between your toes or anything like that?"

"No. Nothing that has bothered me. But I have had an itch on my knee ever since I got on the plane in Peru."

The doctor examined the itchy spot. It wasn't even red, but he probed down a little and then stood up thoughtfully.

"Were you any place you might have gotten a spider bite?"

"When we stopped in Peru and climbed the mountain to see the ruins, we got into a lot of brush."

"I think that might be the thing. This lump could just be infection from that bite that has settled in the lymph gland. I'll give you an antibiotic and that should take care of it. If it doesn't go right away, you let me know."

Dev was still weak and got dizzy if he went without food very long, but he couldn't eat very much. It would be several days before we had the results of his tests. That evening, he called Gayle.

The account of their first meeting was written in her journal:

"Devro came home March 26, 1977, Saturday night about 10:00. I purposely stayed in Ogden for that weekend because I felt uneasy about seeing him. I also didn't want to appear too forward, and I didn't want to expect him to come and see me and then be let down. Later, I was very glad I had made that decision. He called me on Monday. He sounded quite weak and didn't have much to say. I wanted to impress him and build him up a little, so I tried to sound as excited as possible. He asked when I would be coming home and I told him the next Friday. He then asked if he could come to see me, and I told him of course he could.

"Wow! I couldn't wait for that week of school to end. I wanted to see him so bad, yet I was very scared to face him. I was afraid that I might have changed in my appearance for the worse. I started imagining all sorts of things until I believe I was a nervous wreck. When I got ready, I waited and waited and waited until Devro finally called at 10:00 P.M. He said one of his companions had dropped by to see him and he couldn't get him to leave. He told me he would be down in half an hour. I felt so scared, I hoped he would never come. But when he came, I felt so relieved to see him. I answered the door and in about two seconds he was hugging me. I could tell right then that I had grown about two inches. He didn't give me a kiss. He walked into the family room and sat down and we just looked at each other without saying a word. It seemed to be a very uncomfortable situation, but it wasn't at all. I just wanted to look at him. He asked if I would like to go to general conference with him that Sunday and I said yes.

"After that, we dated on weekends without seeing each other during the week because of my school in Ogden. I was trying really hard to finish with good grades.

81

But sometimes Devro would get a job hanging doors in Ogden or near there and would surprise me by coming to see me during the day. Once he came in the morning. He rang the doorbell of the apartment where I lived with several other girls, and we thought it was just our roommate who stayed out late and sometimes forgot her key, so my friend opened the door. I was in the bathtub at the time, and very innocently walked out into the living room with my bathrobe on and curlers in my hair. There sat Devro on the couch. I just about died! He had never seen me in curlers before. But he didn't seem shocked; he just gave me a big hug and a kiss. I hurried and tore out my curlers.

"And once after coming to see me in Ogden, Devro got into his car next to mine and mouthed the words 'I love you,' and blew me a kiss. It was the neatest thing I had ever seen him do."

Watching Devro discover Gayle's many talents was very interesting for me. I had never decided in my mind that Gayle would be the girl he would marry. I knew she had wonderful qualities of faithfulness, dependability, chastity, and all the things a mother looks for in a girl for her son to marry. But people are attracted to each other for many and varied reasons, and for a mother or anyone else to try to pick a mate for anyone, least of all her only son, would be ridiculous.

Each night they went out together, Dev would come home with more talk of some new talent of Gayle's that he had become aware of.

"Mom, do you know Gayle can sing? I was sitting by her at their home evening tonight and when we sang—she can really sing."

Another night: "Mom, Gayle cooked dinner for me tonight and she can really cook."

"Dev, are you beginning to like Gayle?"

"I've always liked her, Mother. I love her, but I don't know if it's the kind of love you marry for. Heavenly Father hasn't told me that. And..."

"Yes?"

"Well, she has the most beautiful hair . . . and her eyes—I could eat her for her eyes."

"I wouldn't if I were you."

"Wouldn't what?"

"Eat her for her eyes."

"Oh, Mom—you and your sense of humor. You know what I mean."

"You mean she has beautiful eyes, but you seem hesitant. What don't you like?"

"Well, she's not really beautiful, not like some of the girls I've gone with."

"How do you mean that? You mean she hasn't as nice a figure?"

"Oh, no. She was kind of straight up and down when I left, but she's filled out in all the right places."

"I know. Then what is it you don't think is beautiful?"

"I don't know."

I smiled. He really seemed puzzled. I knew more about what he meant than he did. Gayle was the kind of girl who wasn't strikingly beautiful, but had an inner softness, a realism that grew more beautiful as you knew her. Hers was the kind of beauty that would glow even more as she grew older, and when such a girl fell in love . . . I smiled, knowing there was lots in store for Mr. Devro Sealy. But there was no use telling him this; it would just get him arguing with me to convince himself. Instead, I asked, "Maybe you think she looks too plain in her jeans? When she helped you wash the car the other day and she had her hair in pigtails, I thought she looked like your little sister."

"Oh, no, Mom, I love her in her grubbies. She looks so cute. I like her in jeans."

"You don't like her dressed up?"

"Yeah, but—I don't know."

Then, one night, after Dev had been on a job near Ogden and I knew he had seen Gayle, he came home obviously upset. He took my hand and pulled me away from Loni and her friends in the kitchen and took me to his room.

"Something is the matter with me, Mom."

"I thought you were upset. What has happened?"

"I don't know, Mom. I don't know what is happening to me. I feel as if something terrible is going to happen, the worst thing that has ever happened to me."

"Like what?"

"I don't know. In the mission field I had a feeling like this, and I was afraid something would happen to Dad before I got home. I finally decided it was just Satan trying to discourage me. But now I have the same feeling, only I don't think it is Dad."

"Has it got something to do with your future?"

"Yes, I know it has."

"Let's talk about your future. Do you want to go away to school?"

"No, I don't want to live in a dorm or away from home. I've been away long enough. I don't want to cook for myself or wash or—."

"Do you want to drive to school from here?"

"No. I've had enough of that."

"Do you want to get married and take a wife with you?"

"I don't know." He began to pace up and down the room. "I think I do. I didn't think I would for a long time, but maybe I do."

"Is it Gayle?"

"I don't know. I wish I could get an answer to my prayers."

"What does Gayle say?"

"I stopped in to see her today and asked her what she thought about us, and she just looked at me and said, 'Don't worry, Dev, everything will be all right.' "

I smiled, thinking what a wise girl Gayle was. To Dev I said, "Would you like your father to give you a blessing? Maybe that would calm you and help you to be less confused."

"I would like that, Mom."

So we went upstairs to Milt's room. He hadn't been feeling well and had gone to bed early in the evening. I woke him and he gave Dev a father's blessing. Then he sat on the bed and talked to his son for a few minutes.

"Dev," he said, "maybe you are trying too hard to get your answers. You know, when I have a problem and I pray for answers, after praying I go out and work really hard and try to get the problem off my mind. Then some little thing happens and there's the answer."

So Dev decided to go out of town on a big job he had scheduled and to try to forget about decisions for a while. When he came home, he still had his fears, but he had decided to put Gayle through some tests while he waited for the answer to his prayers. He had a date with her that night.

I was in the kitchen sewing when Dev came home from the date.

"You know, Mom, tonight Gayle wore a long dress and her hair was so beautiful and, you know, Mother, Gayle is really beautiful."

"I know, Dev."

"No, Mother, you don't understand. She really is beautiful, not just for me but she's beautiful for anybody to see."

"I know, Dev."

"I think she's really changed. She's beautiful. I see her eyes before me all the time."

"A girl does change, Dev, when she falls in love. She gets more beautiful because she glows from within."

"Do you think she's in love, Mom?"

"Don't you?"

"Yes, I guess she is." He said the words thoughtfully, with a smile on his face; he wasn't conceited, just confident and happy. Then his expression changed to a troubled look. "Yes, but I've got to be sure this is what Heavenly Father wants for both of us."

Before the next weekend Dev came to me and invited me to go downtown with him.

"Would you like to go with me to pick out a setting for my diamond?"

"Thinking of making yourself a ring?" I teased.

He smiled. "Yeah. Want to help me decide?"

"If you want me, that's where I want to be."

That was a great day, being with my son, sharing this secret with him. I couldn't help thinking how different this day was compared to the one when he had bought the diamond. His tests had all been negative; his dizziness and illness were gone. Now here he was, seriously thinking of marriage, and he hadn't been home even a month. It was as if some strange, sweet spirit were pushing him faster than he wanted to go.

"Four-year college boy, huh?" I teased.

"I know, but I'll get my schooling. I'm flying up to Colorado to check into their courses. Gayle's sister and brother were down last week and invited me to check it out. If I fly, they'll let us stay with them."

"Us?"

"I thought I would take Gayle with me. Dad has arranged an inexpensive flight. We'll just stay a couple of days. They'll show me around the college. It's kind of part of the test. I want to see Gayle in family surroundings, just to see how I feel about her when we're together more than on a date."

"Be careful of the girl's reputation." I was teasing, but Devro was suddenly serious.

"You think I won't be? I don't want any hint of anything that might put her in a wrong light."

"Of course not—I can see that. Don't be so touchy."

"It's serious, this marriage stuff. If that's what it is. I think this will be the best test. If we come home and I still think this way, then I'm going to give her the ring, but I won't take it with me. I'll wait until we're home again before I say anything. More than anything, Mom, I don't want to hurt her."

"You're going to test her all the way, aren't you."

"Yes, I was afraid maybe she was too sweet to be a good mother."

"What do you mean, too sweet?"

"Well, I used to think the most important thing in a

wife was that she was obedient to her husband, but in the mission field I added a new dimension. I saw whole families, wonderful kids, strong in the Church, even when their father wasn't, and in every case they had kind of a mean mother. I had to find out if Gayle was strong enough to be the mother of my children."

"And is she?"

"She is. I found out the other night at her house. Her little brother got out of hand. She told him to do something and he wasn't going to do it, and boy, she was firm. She didn't raise her voice, she just looked at him, was firm, and waited. He obeyed. She's strong enough to be a good mother."

"And now you think Gayle is the one?"

"I think so, but I haven't gotten an answer yet. I don't know why I haven't gotten an answer."

"Have you had a 'no' answer?"

"No. Everything seems to be all right."

"Then why not go ahead, unless you have strong opposition or confusion?"

"Is that what you think I should do, Mother?"

"You're trying to get me to say one way or the other so you can have a wonderful time arguing with me, aren't you?"

"Well, maybe . . ."

"No, dear. This is your decision. I love Gayle. I have always loved her and I'll go on loving her even if you don't decide to marry her. I love you too, but I'm not wise enough to know if you are right for each other. I'll sit tight and do what you want me to do."

11

The crisis had passed. Gayle would live, at least for now. She had improved—very little, but it was a sign of progress. Dev called before I went to bed that night.

"Mom? Gayle seems better tonight. When I went in to see her she told me she wanted to die; she felt her hair and all the instruments and she thinks she looks ugly. I told her she was beautiful and she wasn't going to die, so she just had to hurry and get well and get out of that bed."

"That's what she needs, a strong, positive attitude."

"Nothing is going to be negative around her anymore. If she has another calling, Heavenly Father is just going to have to take her because I'm praying for healing, for her to be blessed."

"You sound better tonight. Have you had some sleep?"

"Yes, I slept for several hours, off and on. I helped bless the man in the other critical bed. He's had a bad night."

"You're everybody's strength, so get some sleep so you will be able to be of help and not let negative thoughts get to you."

"I will. I'm going to have prayer with Gayle now and then we will get to sleep. I just called for the report on Skyler. Jean went down to see him tonight, so I'll go in the morning."

"Vicki is going to see him in the morning too. I'll go tomorrow night."

"You've all been great."

"Don't worry about anything here; we'll keep you informed. Everything will be all right."

I climbed into bed still thinking about Dev and Gayle. What a storybook romance they had had. I remembered the day I went to the airport to pick them up when they got home from Colorado. I could see they were tired, but they talked all the way home. Dev and I dropped Gayle off at her place first, then drove home together.

"Well," I said when we were alone, "did she wear well in a family atmosphere?"

"Did she? She's a sweetheart, Mom. It's going to be Gayle unless I get a 'no' answer from Heavenly Father. No one is better with children than Gayle. You should see her with her sister's children. We took them everywhere with us. And they are the sweetest little girls."

That week Linda and I went to a movie, *The Slipper and the Rose*. I knew it was the story of Cinderella, and I didn't especially want to see that again, but there wasn't really any other choice, so we went ahead.

How delightfully surprised we were! Cinderella with a new twist, so light, romantic, funny, and uplifting. We left the theater walking just a little above the ground. And so it was that when Saturday came and Milt and I were leaving town for a day, Dev said, "Tonight I'm going to give Gayle her diamond, Mother. But I've got to think of some special way. It's got to be really good. I've got reservations for our favorite restaurant, but I want to give her the diamond in a special way."

"I wish I could help you, Dev, but you kids always think my ideas are stale, so I've quit thinking them up."

"I'm going downtown shopping now, but I can't think what I want to get. I guess I'll find something."

"Oh, there is one thing you might like. Linda and I loved the show *The Slipper and the Rose*. If you want to sort of float on air with a romantic mood, that's the show to see."

"A show would make us too late."

"Just an idea."

Thinking about this part of their romance now, as I sat alone in the house, I opened Gayle's book of remembrance again, hoping to find out how she had written up that special engagement night.

"On April 30th, a Saturday night, Devro took me to a show called *The Slipper and the Rose*. It was about Cinderella but with unanimated characters. Cinderella happened to look quite a bit like me. After the show I was on cloud nine, and even though it was a fairy tale, I hoped it would someday happen to me. Then Dev took me to our favorite restaurant; it was our favorite because that was where I had fallen 'for sure' in love with Devro. We went in and took off our shoes and sat in the Japanese booth. Devro, for some reason, acted a little nervous. He was cold during the movie and said, after the meal was served, that he wasn't hungry. Devro usually was never cold, and he was always hungry. We had our favorite meal, chicken teriyaki, and then after it had all been cleared away, Devro took out a silver slipper with a note inside. It said, 'Champ . . . take my hand for eternity.' He left me reading it and went outside for something. I felt so scared because I wasn't sure what was happening. I started to cry a little and to laugh a little. All I knew was that I was very happy.

"When Dev came back into the restaurant he was carrying a big box. He asked me to close my eyes. Then after a minute he said, 'Okay, you can look.' There stood a beautiful doll dressed in pink, just like Cinderella, standing on a music box. She started turning around as the music box played, and there on her hand was a beautiful golden diamond. Devro took the ring off the doll's hand and placed it on my finger. Then I started to really cry. I scooted over into his arms and we sat there hugging each other. That was one of the happiest moments of my life. Devro didn't even ask me to marry him; he already knew what my answer would be. That night we first went to my parents' home and I found out Devro had asked for my father's permission earlier in the day. So I told Mom and we were all so happy. Mom and Dad were in bed and I just ran in and jumped on them. What was funny was that Devro followed me in, and I think he was very embarrassed when he realized.

"Then we went to Devro's parents' house and showed them. We went to Aunt Claudia and Uncle Roger's next, Neal and Judy's, Aunt Dona and Uncle Andy's, and Dev had to tell Kevin. We went to Linda and Dale's, Vicki and Richard's—getting everybody up to tell them and show off my diamond. It was about 4 A.M. when we finally got home. It was the most wonderful night because we loved each other so much. After a week of thinking about when we should set the date, we finally decided on the seventh day of the seventh month of the seventy-seventh year. I secretly planned the special once-in-a-century date. But Dev soon figured it out. I had only two months to get my wedding ready—only one month, really, because I wouldn't be out of school until June 8."

I stopped reading to think about those happy moments. Then I smiled and laughed out loud, remembering how Dev, who had never been interested in talking about sex, suddenly wanted to know all about everything. We had always been very open in our home, discussing details of whatever the children were curious about. But Dev had always figured he knew all the essentials, so he had never asked many questions. Now, suddenly he wanted to know all about marriage—much more than the birds and the bees ever told. He was sincere, sweet, and easy to talk to. He asked every question he could think of to ask. Then, to my surprise, the next night he brought Gayle up, sat her down in a chair in front of me, and told me to tell her everything I had told him.

I had laughed about it at the time, but as their relationship progressed I decided that that was the secret of their perfect communication: they were always on the same level; each wanted to know what the other knew, and from the very beginning their secrets were shared.

Once they were engaged, there were no more tests. They did everything together when Gayle was home from school, but when she had to go back to college, Dev was fidgety and unsure. He would go back to thinking about how he had decided not to be married for a long time, and wondering what he was doing by getting married so young.

"Marriage is a real responsibility. I'm not sure I'm ready for so much responsibility," he would say. But then Gayle would come home, he would pick her up, and all the doubt would rush away.

What a happy girl Gayle had been then! Her quietness had suddenly blossomed into loveliness and an outpouring of her personality, and she was always thinking of Devro more than herself. I read on in her journal:

"I graduated from Weber with honors. Dev's mom made me a dress, the first dress anybody else ever made for me. And she and Dev's dad, Dev, Loni, and my parents attended my graduation. Now I could get on with my wedding plans.

"The wedding reception was in blue and white with colored daisies and roses. The whole night turned out gorgeous! But first I have to tell about the beautiful day in the temple when Devro and I were sealed. As soon as we got inside the temple, the brides were dressed and prepared. I was very nervous until I went through the doors of the temple. Then the calmest, most beautiful feeling came over me. I felt as though I were dreaming the whole thing. My body was numb and I couldn't believe that I was real. It seemed as though my body was a robot, programmed to do everything, but my mind was saying, 'What's going on?' Then Devro and I met and we were escorted to an elevator and told to stop on a certain floor. We got off and were escorted to a sealing room. We sat on a special seat in front of the altar and both our fathers sat across from us in upholstered chairs. They were to act as witnesses. Our mothers sat on each side of us. I must mention that before we were taken into the sealing room, we were taken to the celestial room to sit and ponder over what was about to take place. Devro and I sat and looked at each other and I felt so good; tears came to my eyes because I was so happy. He talked a little and expressed his love for me and I did the same. Then Devro asked to see my engagement ring, saying, 'I don't want to fumble around on the most important day of my life.' He practiced hooking the wedding band to my engagement ring and then after a minute said, 'I've got it.' Then a kind lady stepped in and had us come to the sealing room.

"Robert L. Backman, who was later made a General Authority, began talking. He talked about our roles as husband and wife. I remember him saying to me, 'If Dev comes home to a wife who has curlers in her hair and the children are crying and the house is a mess, don't expect him to act like the special husband you've always dreamed about. If you do your best, your relationship will stay happy and will grow.' He also counseled us to continue with our dating, to set aside a night every week for each other. He told us to find time to be together, to take an interest in each other's work and interests. This great man had so many wonderful things to say to us; sometimes while sitting there I wondered if I was worthy enough to have this beautiful experience. The Spirit was very strong while he talked to us. Dev held my two hands in his the whole time. Then we were asked to kneel at the altar holding hands. There were beautiful mirrors on each side of us. Devro's eyes were so inspiring, so wonderfully blue; I could not look at anything but his eyes. His hand securely held mine, and when the Spirit became stronger in my heart, I knew it was doing the same in his heart because of the way he looked at me.

"That day was so wonderful, I wanted to be the perfect wife for Devro. I wanted him to have everything. I wanted to make him happy throughout all eternity. I wanted to bear his children and I wanted to go through pain and hardship with him. I just wanted to be with him forever.

"Following the temple ceremony, pictures were taken outside. I had to put on my veil and get ready. Several little ladies plus my mother were pinning my veil on my head. I was so fussy because I knew I would be looking at those pictures the rest of my life. Finally Mom and I got ready and left the temple to meet everyone on the temple grounds. There Devro stood in a white suit trimmed with blue suede, waiting for me. He was so very good-looking I grabbed hold of his arm and he turned to me and squeezed me. It seemed as though all of our relatives were there—everyone with a camera in hand.

"But we had to wait for the photographer. Nearly an hour passed and he still wasn't there. I was so embarrassed. I didn't know what I would do if we didn't have some really nice pictures of us after our marriage. Finally he did come and all went well.

"Next on our schedule was the wedding breakfast. The most memorable things that happened there were the words of advice given to Dev and me. My father told us to always take time to be together—to find common interests and work on them together. I remember expressing my thoughts, and all that came to my mind was that I should tell the unmarried girls there that everything was worth working for to have a temple marriage. I thought of all the depressing moments I had gone through when I was single, and I knew they were all worth going through if a temple marriage was the final result. Judy gave a cute word of advice. She said that it is always best to have supper ready when your husband gets home, and if you can't have it ready, set the table. That way he is more willing to wait because it looks as though you are more prepared. I thought that was funny but very smart!"

I closed Gayle's journal. That was the last entry into that book. What would happen now? I asked myself. Would she get well and fill up the rest of the empty pages of her journal? Or was her mission somewhere else more important? She was so young to go through so much. I thought of Dev staying beside her in the hospital night and day, never leaving except to shower or drive to Provo to see their son. In a way, it was harder on Dev than Gayle—he was so helpless—yet, it was Gayle trying to hold on, to get well for Devro. How much did she feel? How much of this nightmare of pain would she remember when she came home?

I had been to their apartment to water their plants, and I had had a wonderful warm feeling, as if Gayle had just left for a little while and would be back soon. The spoons, ready for the dessert she had been planning to serve her Beehive girls, were still on the countertop. The dessert in the refrigerator had spoiled and I had had to throw it out. The chairs in her front room were still in the same position she had put them in for her class. She would come back: we had to believe that, and to pray for her. Prayer was all we had. The doctors were doing all they could, but nothing seemed to turn out the way they anticipated... not even yet, and it had been two weeks.

12

While the fight for life went on in the hospital, Father's Day appeared on the calendar. As ill as Gayle was, she communicated to her mother what she wanted Devro to have for Father's Day. The rest of us, as we thought about shopping for our own husbands and fathers, couldn't help thinking about Devro. To help him realize what we were all feeling for him, Judy and Neal invited him to dinner and Linda bought little Skyler a pair of blue booties. Vicki took the booties to the hospital and put them on Skyler and took his picture in them. Then she made a little book containing messages from Skyler to Daddy Devro. The girls took the booties and the book to the hospital to give them to Devro.

Dev was thrilled. After he read the messages and looked at the pictures, he took them in to show them to Gayle. Linda and Vicki were allowed to go in with him. When they told Gayle the little booties had been on Skyler's feet, she lifted them to her lips and kissed them. She was so weak that it was difficult for her to get her arms up that high. Her eyes were bandaged and she couldn't see, but when she kissed the booties and put them to her cheek, we knew she understood.

Little Skyler, like his mother, was still having his bad days, and we were still uncertain as to what Heavenly Father had planned for him. Gayle had been through so much to give her little son life that we hoped Heavenly Father wouldn't take him from her. But she was still so critical herself that we didn't know if she would live to be with him if he did live. The doctors didn't give us much hope, except to tell us that Gayle's youth was a big factor in her favor and there wasn't anything wrong with her that couldn't change and be all right if she would just turn that corner and start healing. Whatever the outcome, I felt Devro and Gayle were being prepared for a great mission. That thought kept hanging on stronger than any other.

In the meantime, life was going on outside the hospital. Dev had come to the point where he really needed to leave the hospital sometimes to pay bills and make calls about his business, but he didn't want to leave because he was afraid he might be needed to make decisions or to sign papers. And he worried that Gayle would call for him and he wouldn't be there. Finally he decided to get himself a beeper to wear so we could always contact him. I went up to the hospital to sit with Gayle the day he arranged for the beeper service. She was pretty quiet that day, so I talked to the people in the waiting room as they came and went.

There were so many people with so many problems. I listened to their anxieties and watched as they came and went. Almost everyone's problems were solved in a few hours, a few days, or a couple of weeks. But the problems in Gayle's room seemed to go on and on. Through it all, Dev was positive in his thinking and in the way he treated his sweet Gayle.

Then one morning, when I went to visit, Dev was really discouraged. He was usually so positive in his thinking that not even the doctors' negative reports could get him down, but this morning it was apparent that he was unnerved inside.

"What is it, Dev?"

"One of the doctors told me that if Gayle doesn't rally soon, we might have to make a decision to shut the machines off. I'm not going to do that."

"You shouldn't have to—that's not in your hands."

"The doctor seems to think it might be."

"Did he say that?"

"Not in so many words, but he said she couldn't go on this way indefinitely. Of course, I know that."

"Has she had a bad day today?"

"Yes. She has had to have more blood, and..." He paused as if his mind were moving rapidly over too much, then went on to a new subject. "I was in with Gayle a little while ago, and the doctor wanted me to leave while he put another tube in her lungs, but Gayle wanted me to stay. So I just told him that it wasn't up to him or anyone else in the room whether she lived or died, so to just go ahead and do what he had to do and I would stay."

"I can see that you've had a bad day yourself."

"Yes, I have. If only I knew what is happening. It's so hard to just stand still wondering what to do."

"I know," I said, and I couldn't help thinking that it seemed as if all I knew how to say was "I know."

Dev couldn't leave Gayle that day, so I left early and went to see Skyler, and then I planned to go to the temple again. Skyler startled me; he seemed so much weaker. I rubbed his little feet and sang to him, but he didn't open his eyes this time, though there was some evidence of response. The nurse explained that he was on a relaxant to keep him from fighting the respirator and to help him save his strength. But I felt there was something more than that wrong. A fear began to tighten inside me, and I was glad that I had planned to go to the temple.

I left the temple feeling better, feeling the same calmness I had experienced before. Everything would be all right. All I had to do was hold on until we knew the will of our Father in heaven.

I went home and did a day's work—hard, physical work. It made me feel better to be tired physically. Then, as the evening came and I knew Dev would be having prayers with Gayle, I called the hospital to check with him before going to bed. His voice was tired and tight.

"I'm worried about Gayle tonight, Mother."

"Is she worse?"

"Different. Her charts are about the same, but the nurse called me in a little while ago because she couldn't get Gayle calmed. They had given her a sedative, but when I went in she was just twisting her sheets in her hands and she was so troubled. I talked to her and she calmed down a little. I sat there and kissed her and told her I loved her and she settled down. But it didn't last; when I thought she was asleep I went out of her room, and in just a little while the nurse came for me again. She was doing the same thing again. I said, 'Gayle, what's the matter, honey?' Then she formed the word *baby* with her mouth, and I said, 'Your baby?' and she nodded."

"Dev, was she worried about Skyler?"

"I thought she was thinking back to before he was born, so I explained the whole thing to her again—how she has had the baby and everything. But that wasn't it. She knew she had had the baby. She's worried about him."

"I've been worried about him too, Devro. But I know Heavenly Father loves him even more than we possibly can."

"I know, Mother."

There it was again: *I know*. I talked to Dev a little more, then let him go so he could try to get some sleep. I wanted to try to get some sleep myself, but I wasn't counting on it. Late that night the telephone rang again, and I knew I wasn't the only one who wouldn't sleep. The call was from Vicki, who was at the hospital with Skyler.

"Mother?"

"Yes, Vicki."

"I didn't wake you, did I?"

"Not a chance. What's wrong?"

"If you aren't too tired, Mother, I would like to drop by and talk to you on my way home."

"I'm not too tired. Come on!"

I hung up, but even before she came I knew what she wanted to talk about. She had been with Skyler and she was worried.

I showered and was slipping into a robe when I heard Vicki open the back door. One look at her face told me what she had been through watching that little boy.

"Mother, he looks so bad. If little Skyler can't be healed, oh, Mother, I don't want to see him dwindle away little by little and watch him suffer. If he can't live, why can't he go peacefully? He's such a cute little boy, and he tries so hard."

The tears dropped freely down Vicki's face as she talked. She had always been tenderhearted about babies. I knew what these daily trips to the hospital had taken from her in time and emotion.

"You think he's worse, don't you."

She nodded.

"I feel the same way. When I saw him this morning I felt that he was going down."

"What can we do?"

"Just what we have been doing: pray, pray, and pray some more."

"Dev calls for a report every few hours, but he hasn't seen Skyler yesterday or today because he can't leave Gayle long enough to make the trip from Salt Lake to Provo. The reports they give him don't tell the whole picture, Mother. If Dev saw him, he would know."

"Maybe he knows anyway. Dev has that extra sense about those he loves—and Gayle does, too."

"But we've got to do something about little Skyler."

"Maybe by morning we'll know more. He belongs to Heavenly Father more than he belongs to us; surely, loving him so much, Heavenly Father will take care of his little early son. Surely he won't let him suffer without reason."

"Poor little guy. He's already lived a lifetime in fifteen short days."

Vicki left, wiping her eyes, and I knew she had been crying a lot.

As I went upstairs to get into bed, I thought about Devro driving back and forth between hospitals and about the terrible turmoil he was going through. My mind went on churning, over and over, with pictures, images, and vague thoughts. Over and over I saw myself trying to comfort Devro, and knowing that in the end Devro would be the one to comfort me. This was his family, and he was in charge. Yet in my half-awake and half-asleep dreams, I seemed to realize that both Skyler and Gayle would leave us. The thought hit me so hard that I sat up in bed. It slipped away again as I prayed, but by morning I knew that at least Skyler would definitely leave us. He was close to the end.

I called the hospital in the morning, and the doctor's report supported my feelings. Skyler was very weak, and the doctor's only instructions were to make him as comfortable as possible.

I called Devro, and the sound of his voice, rather than his words, told me he knew something was the matter.

"Are you going to be able to visit Skyler today, Devro?"

"I can't leave Gayle, Mother." His words were a little sharp.

"Don't worry, I'll call Vicki and see if she is going to see him. If she can't, I will."

"Thanks, Mother."

"If Vicki can be with Skyler, do you want me to come up to be with you and Gayle?"

"Yes, Mom. Thanks."

I hung up and dialed Vicki's number. She was already up.

"I'll go be with Skyler, Mother. You go to Devro."

"All right, dear, I will. He's really upset, I can tell, even though he's still in control. But there's something about his voice that warns me. Gayle has been so long without a change now, I think he's afraid that when the change comes it won't be a good one. He has to be with her."

"One request, Mother: If Dev can't be with Skyler, and the time comes when we know, ask him if he doesn't mind if I hold Skyler in my arms, just once, like a real baby."

"I'll ask him, dear. Vicki, thank you."

As I hung up I wanted to sit down and cry, cry until all the hurts were washed away, but again, this wasn't the time. Dev had said to me one day as we sat talking in the waiting room, "People say I'm so calm. Little do they know I would like to run through the hospital screaming. I would, too, if it would do any good." He had said those words as if he were talking about the weather, but I knew he meant them. How would he take the news about Skyler? How would I tell him? How much did he already know?

I arrived at the hospital, and one look at Devro told me he hadn't slept at all. There was a nervousness in his eyes. He knew more than he wanted to talk about, I was sure of that. He sat down stiffly, and I sat beside him.

"Dev," I said quietly, "Skyler is sleepy. He's tired, and he needs to go to sleep."

Dev let out a long, deep sigh, and the stiffness went out of his back. His words were tender and full of desperation at the same time.

"I know, Mother. I know."

"Dev, I think Skyler needs his father to tell him he can go to sleep."

"I can't leave Gayle, Mother."

"I know, Dev. Vicki has gone down to be with him. I'll go too, if you don't need me here. Vicki asked that if you can't be with him, could she be the one to hold him in her arms, just for a little while?"

Dev's shoulders heaved with another deep breath, then he sat up straight. "Mother, that's what I want to do. I want to hold him in my arms."

"My car is outside full of gas."

"We could come right back, couldn't we?"

"As soon as you want to."

"I'll talk to Gayle and see what she thinks."

Dev went in to see Gayle and Jean, and came out a few minutes later saying, "Gayle says she wants me to go."

He took my arm then, and we went downstairs together and out into the parking lot where my car was waiting. As he backed the car out and started toward the freeway, he said, "Mother, I want to get a little blue blanket to wrap him in. I want to hold him in a little blue blanket the color of his eyes."

We met Vicki at the Utah Valley Hospital intensive care nursery. After we scrubbed, Dev walked over to Skyler's little waterbed and spoke to his tiny son cheerfully. Skyler recognized his father's voice, and he opened his pretty blue eyes. It was the first time he had opened them for quite a while.

Dev took the white blanket the nurse offered him and held his son in his arms, instruments and all. He talked to him and told him how much he loved him; then he blessed him and told him he could go to sleep if he wanted to. He could go back to his Heavenly Father again where he could rest from this time of hurting. Then he let Vicki hold him for a little while, and as we watched the machines that recorded his heartbeat we knew he was getting weaker.

Now it was my turn. Dev went out into the hall to lie down for a minute on the couch while I stayed with Skyler, and Vicki went home to her children. I promised to call her if we needed her. I talked to my grandson for a little while and then went out in the hall to be with Dev. He was resting quietly on the couch; I thought he might possibly be asleep, so I sat down softly. He moved a little and I knew he wasn't asleep, but he didn't say anything.

I thought back to the day when he and Gayle had announced they were having a baby. They had anticipated only happiness. I remembered that Milt had prided himself for thinking ahead: excited as they were when they left on their honeymoon, Milt knew how crazy they both were about babies, so when he went to work that day he told the bookkeeper to fix their insurance for children in the immediate future.

But they hadn't started their family immediately. They had been married almost six months before Gayle got pregnant. By that time they had had a honeymoon, bought a new house, moved into an apartment while they finished their new house, and both of them had worked hard: Dev laying floors and putting in a sound system, and Gayle decorating. They had fixed up their basement to give karate lessons to a group of young boys. Then a few months later they had decided to sell their new home and build another one. But that Christmas, their first Christmas, they had spent in their own new home. I could see them now as they sat together at the Christmas party with the family, anxious to share their Christmas present with all of us. Gayle was happy and blushing as Devro made the announcement—as if he were about to become the only father on earth. And he was like that. One friend had said, "Gayle and Devro are so darling together. He struts around like he's having the baby, and he always tells her how beautiful she is—even more beautiful now that she is having a baby. I think that's neat."

Yes, that was neat. Little did that sweet couple know it would be so difficult to start their family.

Dev roused a little. He must have been thinking about those times, too.

"You know, Mom, Gayle hardly ever makes a mistake, but she thought Skyler would be a girl. We both did. You know what she said when I told her he was a boy?"

"What?"

"She said she knew she would beat her sisters having the first boy, but she thought it would be her second child."

We were interrupted by the nurse calling Devro to the telephone. I followed him to the door of the nursery where he went to answer, thinking it must be about Gayle. But he came back out quickly.

"That was the doctor, Mother. He said Skyler is almost gone, and he has instructed the nurses to take off all the instruments and clean him up so I can hold him. Come on, Mother, let's go down to the gift shop and see if we can find a blue blanket."

I called Vicki and we rushed down to the gift shop. They had only one blue blanket, and it was the color of Skyler's eyes. We hurried back to the nursery to wrap him in it. The little nurse who had taken care of Skyler so often wrapped him tenderly; there were no instruments now, and the little boy lay peacefully in his father's arms as the nurse led us to a private spot. Dev asked for a stethoscope and then he held his tiny son, talking to him, his voice never faltering, but his tears falling softly on the blue blanket as he cradled him in his arms, listening for his heartbeat as he put his big hand on his son's tiny head. He spoke tenderly and wisely.

"Little Skyler, little son, I love you so very much. I'm so proud to have a son so pure, so perfect, that all you needed was a body. Your mother loves you, little son, and she prepared your little body for you. Skyler, little boy, I will try so very hard to live to be worthy of you, to live a good life, so I can join you someday and have the privilege of being your father in that other life you are going to. Thank you for fighting so hard to stay with me. And Skyler, when you see your Heavenly Father, when you get over there on the other side where you understand more of these things than we do, please help your mother. She's having some problems now and she is so sick. She needs your help, little son. . . ."

While he talked, Dev kissed his little boy over and over until at last he took the stethoscope out of his ears and said in a whisper, "He's gone."

I watched as his spirit left his little body, and it was like a house when the lights have been turned off.

Dev meant to hold his son until the mortician came, but there was an urgent call from Jean about Gayle, and we had to leave. Dev put Skyler's body, wrapped in the blue blanket, in the arms of the little nurse who had taken care of him, and we hurried to the car.

We drove to the hospital in Salt Lake City as fast as the speed limit and good judgment would allow, and Dev, with his eyes full of tears, said, "I'm afraid for Gayle now. I'm afraid she will go too. There is such a close bond between them."

"Let's not cross that bridge until we get to it. She hasn't gone yet."

There was silence between us while we struggled with

emotions and anxiety, and then Dev said, "Mother, Heavenly Father answered one of my prayers."

"Which one, dear?"

"I wanted to be with my son when he passed away, and I was so afraid I would have to leave before he went. I wanted to be with him when he needed me. Heavenly Father granted that request."

We drove on, and I could see that the struggle within him was tearing him apart. I was usually full of words, but couldn't think of anything to say to comfort him. My heart just about broke when he said, with a hint of a groan in his voice, "Mother, I wonder how much Heavenly Father will ask of me?"

Later, we found out that the nurse had held Skyler's body until the mortician arrived to take him, and that Vicki had arrived too late to see what remained of him. All she saw was his little empty waterbed.

The night before, I had felt so strongly that both Gayle and Skyler would go, but now, in the face of Dev's faith and the knowledge that he was head of his house, my fears for Gayle subsided and the calmness came again with the feeling that everything would be all right. As we stepped off the elevator on Gayle's floor, I wondered how Dev would tell her about her baby. Jean and the nurse were there beside her door. It was the nurse who spoke.

"Don't tell Gayle about her baby."

Dev looked at the nurse, and I could see that it pained him to think that she thought he would do anything to hurt his Gayle. How could she say that to him when he needed comfort so badly, and Gayle was the only one who could give it to him? But he would always think of her and what was best for her.

"You won't tell her, will you?"

His expression changed. I could see that he was thinking the same thing I was thinking, yet he didn't say anything. He just looked at her. She went on.

"She's had a very bad day and we've finally gotten her calmed. Don't tell her."

He looked back and I expected him to say something

sharp. How could the nurse know how he and Gayle shared everything, the good and the bad? Gayle would expect him to tell her. But Dev didn't say anything sharp; instead, his expression changed again, and he said, firmly but gently, "I won't tell her unless she asks me."

That was the best he could do. He was trying hard to hold on to himself, not to spill over with what he had just been through. He made himself sound realistically husbandly as he went in and sat beside Gayle, leaned over and put his arm across her shoulders, and said, "I love you, my Gayle."

She formed something with her lips, but he couldn't quite understand. "Say it again, honey."

She moved her mouth again.

"Your baby?"

She moved her lips again, and this time it was definitely: "Skyler."

"Skyler? You want me to tell you about Skyler?"

She moved her lips again. Dev couldn't tell just what she was trying to say, but it was enough to let him know that she knew. He put his face in the pillow beside her and softly cried. And as the tears finally came he felt her face draw closer to him and together they cried for a little while. Then Devro lifted his head and held her close and said, "He's all right now. He's with Heavenly Father, and we will be with him someday."

Gayle formed the words, "I know."

He talked a little more about the celestial kingdom where sweet, innocent babies go, where their Skyler now was, and for each thing he said Gayle formed the words, "I know."

Of course she knew. She let him know it was all right. Now Dev understood the anxiety that had caused her to wring the sheets, her anxiety all day while he was away, and her calmness just before he got there. She became calm after Skyler had passed away.

Jean had been alone with Gayle all day, and she was tired. I looked at her and knew she was about to break. I put my arms around her.

"Oh, Jean, you are so very tired."

I knew the tears were close, and I watched as she crossed the room to take the arm of a friend who had come to see her, and together they walked down the hall. By the time she returned Dev had come out of Gayle's room. He went to Jean and put his arms around her and kissed her.

"It's all right, Mom," he said. "She already knew. I didn't have to tell her. Gayle knew."

We all helped a little with Skyler's funeral, but Dev and Gayle made all the plans and all the decisions. Ill as she was, Gayle was coherent enough to know what was going on and to tell Devro what he needed to know. She had prepared her small son's body, all he needed for this life, and she decided where he would be laid to rest.

Only the family was told about the graveside service for Skyler, but we didn't exclude anyone who wanted to come. The people lined up along the mortuary hallway. There were flowers, lots of flowers, and cards; some of the cards had money inside. There was one card full of dollar bills from the karate students and the teens who loved both Gayle and Dev.

When it was time for the funeral, Dev still hadn't come, even though he had given detailed instructions. He had had to stay at the hospital while the doctors finished some morning tests to see if Gayle would be all right. He finally came running in just in time to take charge of everything.

Milt said the family prayer in the mortuary, and then Devro picked up the little blue casket and carried it out to the waiting car. At the cemetery, he again lifted it out and carried it to the green mound on the side of the hill where Skyler would at last rest.

Dev took his place beside Skyler's little blue casket to speak to us all. The sun was shining, but the wind blew slightly as he spoke:

"First, on behalf of Gayle, she sends her love, her thanks, and her appreciation to everyone. She's doing very well today. She's much better. And she has taken this a lot better than I have. She is very calm about Skyler, and she knows she will raise him. She mouthed the words to me: 'I will raise him.'

"I would like to share with you some of the happiness and joys we have felt these sixteen days we have had our little son, and I would like to read what I believe he might feel about his little time on earth."

Dev had told me he was going to tell about Skyler, so I knew he had somehow found time to write what he was going to read to us now. His voice was firm and strong, and it caught only once in a while, but he didn't cry. As he began to read, I knew he had taken his material from the day-by-day notes the doctor had left on Skyler's bed and from the things he himself had written in his journal. Dev cleared his throat just once and started.

"*June 7, 1978.* Today I left my Heavenly Father, and now I am in the world. I wasn't supposed to come just yet, but I just couldn't wait any longer. After I was born they wheeled me down the hall where my Daddy first saw me. He was so excited it was almost embarrassing. I was taken to a special place with lots of other little babies. I have my own little waterbed to lie on. All the nurses who take care of me are so nice. This is a good place to be. My Daddy is going to see my Mommy now. He tells me how much he and Mommy love me. I'm so happy I chose them as my parents.

"*June 8*. The doctor says my lungs aren't very good, but they will get stronger as I get older. I lost a little weight, too. I'm down to a slim three pounds. My Daddy says my legs are very strong. He is already helping me stretch so I can do karate kicks. My Uncle Kevin says I'm real studly (that means tough). My Mommy is still in bed recovering, but my Daddy tells me about her every day. She always sends plenty of kisses.

"*June 9*. Today has been kind of a rough day. I've been restless, so they gave me a shot to make me rest. My Grandmas and Grandpas come to see me and tell me I'm cute. I squeeze my Grandma Burch's finger when she puts it in my hand. She stays here all night long. My Grandpa

Burch has a special place for me in the family since I'm his only grandson. His eyes twinkle when he looks at me.

"Grandpa Sealy tells me he will make me a rabbit pen and chicken coop. He says he will even let me help. And Grandma Sealy tells me I look just like my Daddy when he was a baby. I sure love my grandparents.

"*June 10*. My Daddy and Bishop Lowe gave me a name today: Devro Skyler Sealy. I go by Skyler.

"*June 11*. My lungs are starting to improve. I feel much better. I opened my eyes today and can see all the wonderful things of this earth. Everyone says my eyes are like my name: sky blue.

"*June 12*. My Aunt Vicki comes to see me every day since my Mommy can't come yet. She sings my own special song. I love to lie and watch her while she sings. She brought me my own little doggie, rubber duckie, and a big teddy bear just my size.

"*June 13*. My Daddy says I have pneumonia. Both my Mommy and Daddy are in Salt Lake now. My Mommy was moved to another hospital. When my Daddy comes to see me, he rubs my back and talks to me. I'm starting to get impatient. There is so much to do. I want to run, play in Richie's treehouse, and climb mountains with Grandma.

"*June 20*. It has been two weeks now, and I should be strong and healthy. My Daddy gave me a special blessing, so that will help me. I feel that many people love me. I am going to fight my very hardest and try to get better today.

"*June 21*. My Mommy is very restless tonight. My Daddy stays with her and calms her. I want so much to get better, but I have almost used all my strength. I have tried to be a good little boy and get better. I feel a special feeling like everything will be all right.

"*June 22*. Today is the happiest day of my life; I have been called on a mission with my Father in heaven. I guess all these worldly things will have to wait. It will be just a little while and I'll see everyone again. I am HAPPY! My Mommy feels good about this call, and she knows she will raise me later in the eternities. My Daddy is holding me while I say goodbye. Mommy and Daddy, I love you. . . ."

Dev continued, "Little Skyler, we love you. Your mama loves you, and we are happy for you.

"We would like to thank everyone who has helped and prayed and been so thoughtful and kind. I say these words in the name of Jesus Christ. Amen."

Skyler was gone. He was at peace with his Heavenly Father, doing the work he had been called to do. He had lived only sixteen days, but his life had touched us all in a way we had never been touched before. Skyler was a part of the family, and his influence would be with us all forever.

13

We were blessed. We had had Heavenly Father's attention more than we understood at the time. Even the financial problems had been taken care of. Not until Skyler had been laid to rest did we know that Dev's insurance policy, which was supposed to pay just enough to cover a normal pregnancy and delivery, had a clause that paid in full, with only a small amount deductible, when the baby was born from an illness such as Gayle had. And, strangely, it also stated that if the baby lived at least fifteen days there was an additional amount to help with the burial if it should die thereafter. Skyler died the morning of the sixteenth day. These were small blessings in the face of such loss, but blessings that couldn't be denied, that kept us aware that Heavenly Father was in charge and meant only to bless, hoping we were strong enough for such blessings as would come from this great loss someday. In the meantime it seemed he was saying, "You see, I'm with you. I'm answering your prayers. Have faith in the rewards that follow the test."

And what a blessing our friends were! The food we needed for relatives following Skyler's services, and so many extra meals besides, had been provided by loving, tender people of the four wards involved with these two young people. And the money friends offered instead of so many flowers helped Dev pay his current bills and eased the pressure he felt toward all his obligations while he stayed in the hospital with Gayle. The thoughtfulness of people was astounding.

At this time, Dev and Gayle were still paying rent on

the apartment they had lived in for two weeks. The rent was coming due again, and I wondered if Dev wanted an out. I spoke to him about it in the hospital.

"Would you like to get rid of that payment and move back into your old quarters at home?"

"No, thanks, Mom. I don't want to give up the apartment. We had a hard time finding one as new and pretty as that one. Gayle loves it. I don't want to give up the apartment just to save money."

"I know how you must feel—it's home."

"And I want a place for Gayle when she is ready."

"Of course. I offered, after talking to your father, just so you would know you're welcome. When she is well enough to go home, she'll still need a long recovery period. She's welcome to come to our place. But that isn't any big thing; your apartment isn't very far away, and we can arrange to help her every day—and you'll be with her at night."

"If she can just get well enough to leave the hospital."

What else was there to do? Looking at her, knowing how ill she was, it was inconceivable that she would ever leave the hospital, and yet anything was possible with the Lord, and Gayle had always been in his hands.

I remembered so well when they had found the apartment. They had decided to sell their home and build another one, but their first home had sold so rapidly that the new home wasn't ready when they needed it. That was when they had moved in with us at our invitation. We lived close to the new home they were building, and apartments were almost impossible to find for such a short time. But as the time drew near, they had reconsidered taking the new home in view of the many other projects they had started. Schooling was difficult enough with their overcrowded schedule, and so, one morning, as the time for Skyler's birth came closer, they had gone out looking for an apartment and quite accidently had found one they both liked that fit their needs and all the furniture and household things they had acquired so rapidly. But that little while they had lived with us—what a blessing!

Our children had always been independent, doing things for themselves. We had never believed in married children living at home, but things were different this time. Devro had finished his weight room, even carpeting the floor and the walls, before he went on his mission. It was a big room, and with the rest of the basement there was plenty of space. The only thing I had down there was a washroom and another kitchen where I did canning and big baking. I didn't use it much now, with only Loni at home, so Gayle and Dev moved in. They confined themselves mostly to Devro's weight room, and came and went without bothering anyone. The times we did have time to be together were very enjoyable. There hadn't been much time after Dev's mission to hear about his activities there, and we needed time to get to know Gayle.

If all the mother-in-law jokes are true, we should have had a lot of trouble, but instead, the time we were together was a good experience. I knew it was for me, but I wondered how Gayle felt. She was always working, always busy. She could slip in and out of the kitchen to fix a meal for Dev when he was in a hurry and never leave a sign that she had been there. Sometimes she helped so much I worried about her.

"Dev, get your wife out of this kitchen. She's been working all day. Take her somewhere."

I remembered asking Gayle, as they moved to their apartment, "Honey, has it been hard on you living here with us?"

She smiled and kissed me. "It's been a vacation. I haven't been nearly as busy as I was in our house. I guess I've taken advantage of the situation, too. I've spent a lot of time just going with Dev. I won't be able to go with him that much when our baby is born."

Gayle was always quiet and didn't say much unless we really took time to get into a conversation with her. She didn't ever push herself or her opinions. She observed a lot. As I told my daughter once, "Linda, this Gayle is something. She hasn't mentioned it, but she watches me and then I see her do things the way I do them. I'm sure it's just out of respect because this is our house."

"I know, Mother. I was at her apartment and she and Devro had put up little signs of things they wanted to improve on during the week. Gayle had listed as one goal, 'to keep my nails filed better.' I wish that was all I had to work on."

"I couldn't get over her with her wedding. When there were objections to what she had planned, she listened and talked about the other opinion, but in the end she just quietly did what she wanted to do without causing any trouble, and the result was beautiful."

"Hasn't she got any faults?"

"I asked her about that the night I had to give a lesson on improving ourselves. She just jumped to answer: 'Oh, I'll say! I have to work constantly to remember not to yell. I made up my mind when I was little that I wouldn't grow up to be a yeller. I've worked on it constantly and I still have to bite my tongue.' " I was shocked, and her husband's mouth dropped open in surprise. Neither of us had ever heard her raise her voice.

There was one thing Gayle couldn't get into the weight room when they moved home. It was her piano. Dev had given her the piano for Christmas—the only Christmas, so far, they had ever had together. Dev was one excited boy that day.

"Gayle, a router... I can't believe it! The very one we looked at." Gayle smiled and ran into his arms.

They opened the rest of their small presents, and then Dev got her coat.

"We're invited to Richard and Vicki's for breakfast. Come on."

They went into Vicki's dining room and there was Gayle's piano with a big ribbon tied on it. Dev showed her the tag.

"Dev—mine?"

"All yours." Gayle just stood there unbelievingly. Then she started to cry. "Don't cry, Champ. I want you to be happy."

"A piano! All my life I've wanted a piano of my own, but I didn't think I would ever get one."

"This one is only part yours. You'll have to give piano lessons to pay off the rest."

How diligent she had been with her piano students! She had made enough money to cover the payment and more.

Gayle, Gayle, Gayle. I couldn't get her off my mind. I had been with her in the hospital all day, and when I got home there was more of Gayle everywhere. In the deep freeze there were packages of strawberries she had put up because Dev liked frozen strawberries and so did she. In the study on the wall was a picture of Gayle standing by a tree looking up at Devro. And there was her piano, once so alive with music. Alive. What I wouldn't have given to see Gayle sitting at her piano right then.

The days wore on—days of worry, hope, searching, fasting, and prayer. The doctors told us that the longer Gayle was in the hospital, the less her chances were of getting well. Dev began to spend a couple of hours a day working while I stayed with Gayle. I watched the struggle within her, watched her try to live and get better. She fell into a coma, and when she came out of it, still so ill, the doctors helped her sit up, hoping her movement would help stimulate her healing. I watched as she forced herself to sit and hold herself up with her arms, trying with all her energy of spirit and determination as the perspiration fell like a shower of water.

Their first wedding anniversary came and Dev bought her a gold necklace and bracelet to match. The nurses had a big cake made and brought punch for everyone. Gayle mouthed the words "thank you" to everything.

The next day Linda called me at the hospital.

"Mother, it just seems as if Gayle is waiting for us to do something to help her. Isn't there anything more we can do?"

"We could hold another fast."

"It doesn't seem right. I told Dale that last night. It just doesn't seem right that a person as good as Gayle should have to go through so much. But you know, Mom, he reminded me that the Prophet Joseph Smith was in jail and suffered those long months, and he was innocent too."

"And our brother Christ. No matter what we suffer, we can't ever go through what he did. Strange, but his sacrifice is more comforting to me now personally than ever before."

And so the days wore on: up and down, encouragement and disappointment. Day after day, Dev and I talked all day, and he and Jean talked at night. There were hours of sleep, but never undisturbed. Phone calls and more phone calls and a constant stream of friends and strangers who called by to give blood. Dev's friend from his old boyhood neighborhood came by and brought him brownies and made him go out on the lawn by the hospital to throw a football for a while . . . and then he stayed to sleep on the floor beside him. Kevin came and talked and tried to get him to take time for a show—and then went home and broke into sobs.

"Mother, what can I do for him? I would tear a wall down with my bare hands for Devro, but this way . . . there isn't anything, and he's being ripped out inside."

But Dev went on giving blessings, comforting those around him, and treating Gayle as if she weren't ill at all. He wasn't pretending, only being realistic and refusing to let anyone be morbid or sad around his lovely wife.

Then one Saturday night, six weeks after Gayle had gone into the hospital, I went to bed praying and fasting and asking the Lord to please bless her, or if she must go to take her beautifully as she had lived and not let her waste away any more. I pleaded and prayed and went to sleep only to let my mind race around the thoughts and events of the past six weeks. I woke as upset about Gayle as I had been about Skyler the day he died.

Have we been holding on to her? I wondered. *Look at the facts. Look at the opportunities the Lord has had to heal her, and everything, even from the beginning, has been "no." Is he trying to show us? Are we too stubborn to see?*

My thoughts were running rampant as Linda and I drove to Salt Lake City around noon to take dinner to Dev. As I talked with him, I realized that his faith was more perfect than mine, that he wanted only what was best according to the will of the Father. Through all of this he had kept his faith strong and knew Gayle would be blessed somehow.

I worked all the next day with a deep feeling of worry about Devro. He was beginning to look bad. He had talked to the doctors and nurses for a long time, and when Jean had come back to take over, he had gone to meet Stan and hang a door they had promised. He hadn't had any sleep. I prayed and asked the Lord to take charge of the situation and not let them suffer any more. Couldn't he see Devro was breaking too? Dev called me from work.

"Dev, you sound so tired. I've got dinner ready; won't you come home and eat and get some sleep?"

"I can't sleep, Mother. I have to go back to the hospital."

"But you need rest. You aren't any good for Gayle when you are too worn out to think. You're dragging—so long under tension and with no sleep—have you eaten anything?"

"No, I can't eat."

"Please come home, Devro. Please."

"I should be there with Gayle . . . I don't know what to do any more."

"Come home. Sleep and then decide."

"The little boy in the bed next to Gayle died, and I have to dedicate the grave."

"When?"

"In the morning."

"Then you will need sleep. I talked to Jean a little while ago and she is worried about you. Come on home."

"I'll see. I don't know."

I was folding clothes when Dev finally came in. One look at his face and I knew he had been struggling harder than he had ever struggled in his life. He was white and drained. He looked like an old man: the light had gone out of his eyes. He passed me and fell on his bed, and the tears came.

"My little son, my little son," he sobbed. "I miss my little boy so much, and my Gayle..." He rolled over, his hand on his head. "I don't know what to do or where I belong any more. On the way home I thought I was going to pass out. I pulled over to the side of the freeway, and my breath just kept going out and not coming in. I thought I was going to die—and I wanted to. I wanted to so bad! Then I knew I would die if I didn't breathe and so I took a breath, but I didn't know where to go. I didn't know where my home was. It isn't in the hospital; that isn't even Gayle anymore... she's another person... I can't find Gayle. The apartment isn't home—Gayle isn't there. So I went to find Skyler's grave, and I couldn't find it."

"Dev, the marker isn't there yet. But Richie is making one with his woodburning set. We'll put it up tomorrow and then the headstone will be there soon."

"I think I found where it is. I felt good there, as if my little son were there."

He turned over and let the tears come again. I put my hand on his back again and tried to tell him how I felt.

"Devro, I wish I could take your hurt away. As a mother who loves you, I would take away all your hurts if I could, but that would probably make me a bad mother, because we need to suffer our own afflictions and receive the blessings and knowledge that come from suffering. If we knew the blessings that follow great affliction, we wouldn't mind the hurt so much."

"If I only knew what to do. I can't think anymore."

"Then try not to think for a while. Look, Dev, it probably won't help anything, but Vicki and I went shopping yesterday, and she bought you some new pants and I bought you a shirt."

I went back to folding clothes and tried to clear my throat. Dev wiped his eyes and nose and sat up. He picked up the new clothes and came to stand beside me.

"Thanks, Mom, and I'll thank Vicki."

"Sure. And I've got some hot soup ready."

"I'll shower."

"I know you need sleep, but if you feel that you can't, why not go to see a movie with me? We can catch a late one." I knew he didn't care about shows or clothes or anything right now, but even in his great distress he was grateful. He knew what we were trying to do, and he had taken the time to thank us. Whether he would go to a show or not was another matter. But somehow I had to get his mind free from the darkness he was going through, even for a little while.

14

Dev did go to the show with me. He called the hospital before we left, during the intermission, and after the movie ended. Being reassured by Jean, he went home and went to bed. I let him wake up in his own good time the next morning. After he checked with the hospital, we went to the funeral of the little boy who had been in the hospital bed next to Gayle. He dedicated the grave, and we got in the car to leave.

"Dev, you have a beautiful spirit. Your prayer was a comfort to the family. Now what about you? I have to drive to Bear Lake and take some things for the family. Why not go with me? We could come back in the morning."

"I can't."

"It would clear your mind. We will come back as soon as you want to. Kevin is there, and—"

"I haven't got a bathing suit."

"We could drop by the store and get one on our way."

He consented reluctantly after checking with the hospital. I knew he had to get some rest, or he would never be able to make it through the next crisis. Whether Gayle lived or died, he had a lot of heartache still coming.

We went shopping, and Dev found a new pair of swimming trunks and a shirt to go with them."

"I shouldn't be buying clothes."

"You haven't had anything for a long time."

"I don't need anything."

"This is my surprise. You know I've never been able to buy things for you. I always wanted to outfit you for college, but you always did everything for yourself. You even bought all your own mission clothes."

"You bought me a new suit when I came home, and you bought my suit for the wedding breakfast."

"Not much to get for a boy in a lifetime—and that's all I've bought for you since you were little."

We were interrupted by the salesclerk, who knew Dev and wanted to know about Gayle. Then we took our packages, got in the car, and headed for Bear Lake. We stopped before we went through the canyon so Dev could call the hospital once more. Reassured again, we drove through the mountains. Dev talked about Gayle all the way.

"I haven't cared about buying clothes since my mission, except clothes for Gayle. It was fun to buy her things. Before we went to youth conference we went to town and bought her two pairs of shoes at once. She was so excited. And that blouse—remember that pretty blouse with lace? We went to the shopping mall one day to get something else, and I saw that blouse in the window. I showed it to Gayle, and she liked it. I made her go in and try it on. As soon as she tried it on, I told the clerk we would take it."

"She made most of her own clothes, didn't she?"

"Everything. And her clothes didn't look homemade."

Dev talked on, and while he was talking about Gayle he seemed happy.

"The important thing about your life together is that you have always made each other happy."

"She makes me happy. I think I make her happy. I think she will tell me if I don't."

I laughed. "Jean says that over and over—'Dev sure has made her happy.' "

Dev kept talking, as if he hadn't heard me. "We talked about everything. There are so many couples who never have a closeness like ours."

He talked until we were rolling into the driveway of our Bear Lake home. From there on, his cousin Kevin took him over. There were only a few hours of sunshine left, but there was time enough for Dev to swim and water-ski and talk to Kevin. After dark Gayle's sister, who had been there a few days with Loni, sat on the dock and talked with Dev about Gayle. I was content; the diversion was doing him good.

We had planned to leave for home after Sunday School, but Dev called and Gayle was all right, so we stayed for sacrament meeting, and that night in the cabin the young people played games. There was laughter and popcorn and all the things we had loved about Bear Lake and being together—except Gayle. But Kevin didn't have a girl with him, so he and Dev were just two buddies again for a little while, and the hurt had a chance to go underneath for a few hours. Dev began to relax a little.

"Why not stay a while in the morning?" Kevin urged.

"Maybe I will, after I check with the hospital, but I've got to be back by noon."

Just before bedtime, in the middle of the last game, the telephone rang. Dev was immediately alert.

"Don't worry, Dev. It's Vicki."

The noise went on, but Vicki's voice was solemn.

"Mother, Jean called from the hospital. Gayle's had a bad day. Her charts are about the same, but she's been very discouraged. Jean doesn't want Dev to know yet. She says she knows he needs rest."

"She doesn't want us to come home?"

"Not tonight. There's nothing immediate, but she says Gayle is tired of it all and so worn out."

"Dear little Gayle. She's been through so much. Shall I have Dev call?"

"Jean said not tonight."

"All right. I think it would be better if he doesn't rush off in the dark. We'll check the first thing in the morning."

I hung up. The group finished their games, and I went to bed wondering what the morning would bring. This was the first time I hadn't reported every little thing to Dev. He always wanted to see it the way it was, to face everything squarely. But for this once, there wasn't anything he could do tonight, and I didn't know what the morning would bring. I would give him a few hours' sleep.

My sleep that night was fitful: I had that old premonition again. But I knew it was time something should change, and I knew Heavenly Father was in charge. Before I was completely awake, and while the cabin was still, the telephone rang. It cut into the silence like a sharp, sudden roll of thunder. Before I could get up I heard Dev's voice.

"Yes? All right, Stan, let me talk to the doctor. Yes . . ."

There was a tightness in his voice, a little catch, and I knew we would be leaving for Salt Lake City right away. I got dressed and threw a few things in my suitcase, gave the family some instructions, talked to Milt, and was ready by the time I heard Dev on the phone again.

"Is this the highway patrol? Yes . . . I understand . . . but I've got an emergency, and I'll be coming through."

Dev, Gayle's sister, and I were in the car in seconds, and Dev took off. We didn't say much, but Dev explained that the doctor had said Gayle was getting really weak and they had done all they could do. There were a few experimental things left, perhaps . . .

"But I told them not to hurt her any more. I wish they had called sooner."

"I could have warned you last night when Vicki called, but I didn't. Jean said to let you rest a little longer, but she was very discouraged yesterday."

"When I left the hospital the other night I felt as if I didn't ever want to come back until Gayle was sitting up on her bed. But I knew I would."

Thoughts raced through my mind—thoughts and memories—and I felt my prayers had been answered. She was going to go without any more waste of her beautiful body. I knew Dev felt the same way.

Dev was a good driver. He stayed just on the edge of the speed limit most of way through the town areas, but picked up speed in between. The road was reasonably free that time of the morning. When we drove up to the hospital entrance, Dev and Gayle's sister got out and ran in while I parked the car. When I stepped off the elevator, Dev was with Gayle. Looking at Jean's face, I knew. Dev came out of Gayle's room, put his arms around me, and cried.

"Mom, Gayle is dying."

"Does she know?"

He nodded. "She knows."

"Is she afraid?"

"No. She wants to do what Heavenly Father wants. She always has."

"But she doesn't want to leave you, does she?"

"No. But I told her she would be with Skyler."

As long as I live I will never forget those hours that followed in the hospital. Dev sat beside Gayle, talking to her of eternity and what their life together would be like when he rejoined her. He gave courage and positive feelings to us all. The family gathered, and as his sisters appeared he would cry a little with each of them, and then he would smile and go in to see Gayle, each time taking a member of the family with him to see her.

In the waiting room there was mostly positive talk. We laughed some, remembering funny things Gayle had said. There was beauty there beyond anything I had ever felt before. We all had a chance to say goodbye to Gayle and to tell her we loved her. She was easing out slowly, beautifully. As night settled in, we bedded down on the floor. Gayle was weak now, and didn't want to see anyone but Devro. Eventually, even Dev fell asleep for a little while. The nurse had promised to wake him toward the end.

Toward morning the nurses woke first Dev and then the rest of us. We stood around Gayle's bed and watched her last response to Dev's touch. The tears slipped quietly down his face now. He hadn't let her see them before, but now her eyes were shut. He held her hand and kissed her cheeks—and softly whispered his goodbyes. She gave a little gasp on her own . . . and then she was gone.

"My Gayle—my bride . . ."

"It is done. Little Gayle, it is done," I breathed softly.

The nurses turned the machines off. There was silence

in the room for the first time. It was like a symbol of the peace that was on Gayle's face.

We cried quietly for Gayle, this sweet girl we had loved so dearly for such a short time in the flesh. Her mother choked and said, "It hurts so much."

"Yes, it hurts so much."

Dev wouldn't leave until he had gone with her body to the funeral home. I was to pick him up there. While we waited, Vicki said, "That short gasp, as if she saw something. I wonder if Skyler came to meet her?"

Dev nodded. "I'm sure he did."

15

*T*he sun was shining when I woke the next morning. Dev had come home with me after riding with Gayle's body to the funeral home. There was a relief in having the decision made. The wondering was over. Gayle was with her son, and thinking of them together in that beautiful hereafter I had only read about and envisioned was more comfort than I had felt since her illness. Dev was the one I worried about now. He had been so brave and strong. How would he feel when he woke up? I talked to Milt a little in the early hours.

"I have felt all along she would leave us," he said as he dressed for work. "I felt it the first night. I don't think I ever doubted it—only hoped."

"Dev came home with me, and we're moving him into the basement today. Is that all right with you?"

"That's fine. He won't want to be alone right now."

"He said the same thing last night. He's afraid we are relieving him of all his responsibilities, but I told him we just didn't want him to be alone and he said he didn't want to be. I think he's grateful that we want him."

"He's been married such a short time. We didn't see him much after his mission."

"He may not be happy here for long, but for now I'm glad he wants to come home."

"He will marry again. He's so young."

"He knows that. He wants a family, and he has great capacity for love. Once his body heals from the shock and he begins to feel again . . ."

"He will never find anyone like Gayle."

"No, but there will be someone Gayle approves of."

The girls called, and Jean. Since Devro wanted to move home, we had all offered to help. Stan and the boys would handle the heavy things, and the rest of us could box and carry.

Dev came upstairs, dressed and ready to work. I was glad to see that the terrible drained look had eased a little. There was still hurt in his eyes, but a newness too. I knew he had been relieved of the darkness of the hospital rooms he had lived in for so long.

I worried about Dev's going into the apartment with everything Gayle had done all around us. But as we entered, the atmosphere seemed to pick him up, and he sort of wandered around looking at everything, talking about this and that as if enjoying the memory. It seemed to be harder on me than it was on him. I hadn't taken time to really cry before, there had been so much pressure, but now the tears flooded my eyes and I had to swallow hard to be able to talk when Dev asked questions. Everything was so perfect, a little house all set up for living, and we were going to pack it all away. I started packing things in the bedroom, but Dev called me into the front room.

"Look, this is the programming Gayle did to teach her class that night. She used the key idea to put over her point. She fed this whole thing into the computer."

"These plants look pretty bad," called Linda from the kitchen. Dev went to investigate.

"Careful of that little one. We bought that on our honeymoon."

"Shall I take them home and see if I can revive them?"

"Yes. I especially want that little one. Gayle knew just how to take care of all her plants."

He talked and talked, showing us one thing after another, from pictures to clothes and trinkets—each one with a history. It hurt to tear into her things that way, but the more it hurt the faster I worked until at last Dev and I had to leave to meet with the funeral director. I left the girls finishing the packing as Dale came with his truck to start the moving.

"I know I should feel worse than I do, sadder," said Dev, as he backed the car out of the driveway, "but I'm happy somehow, as if Gayle was with me."

"I think she is, Dev."

We went into the mortuary to pick out her casket. As we entered a room full of caskets of many styles and colors, Dev looked around and pointed to a white one.

"That's it. That's the one I saw."

"You saw one?"

"Didn't I tell you, Mother? That night I slept in our apartment, just a little while before she died—when I went to get some things and stayed to sleep for a little while. That night I prayed so hard. I wanted to know what Heavenly Father wanted. And I saw in my mind, just as clear as clear, a white casket on the hill beside Skyler's little blue one. It startled me, and I thought that was my answer until I checked with the hospital and found she was better that day. Then I thought it had just come from my troubled worry. But that white one is the one."

The inside of the casket was lined with pink-peach silk.

"We'll color-key everything in white, peach, and blue. Gayle would want everything color-keyed."

Her temple clothes were new and the finest made. We ordered flowers and then went to town to get Dev something to wear. I could tell he wanted something to match, everything the way Gayle would have done it. This was his tribute to her, the only thing we could do for her now—our last public appearance with Gayle.

Dev found a sky blue suit trimmed in rust thread, with a pink shirt to go with it. Then we went home to work on some last-minute details for the newspaper and to meet with Jean for Gayle's history—so many things Dev really didn't want to think about, but knew must be done. I busied myself moving him into the basement.

It was amazing, I thought as I straightened things around to make room, how much these two people had accomplished in a short year. The gospel had led their lives; that was apparent in everything. They had food storage, a lot for such a short time: seeds in little containers all labeled and ready for planting or sprouting, and wheat in plastic containers. I couldn't believe all they had accumulated in furniture and dishes. For a single man Dev had the best trousseau in town. We would tease him about that in times to come.

I worked on the basement most of the night. I had to get Dev's room straightened around so he could find things and would feel that he had a place of his own. People sent things—food, flowers, plants—and many people called. And there were so many for us to call.

The next day was spent getting ready for the viewing and finishing up last-minute details of preparation. We moved quickly; as a family we seemed to be sustained even more than we had been sustained through the hospital ordeal. Gayle's influence was everywhere, and we were all anxious to make this a memorable time, a happy, temporary farewell. We would think about our loss and hurt later.

Then, suddenly, everything was finished and we stood together at the funeral home. We stood there for three and a half hours while people came through as fast as the line would let them. They lined up around the largest room and down the hall and into the street. When the people were finally gone, Dev stood beside Gayle, sleeping so peacefully now, shook his head, and said, "I can't believe this; it seems so unreal."

Later, when he came home we sat by the kitchen table and talked. He seemed to want to talk. One thing he said will always be with me: "Mom, people say how perfect she was and what a good marriage we had, but they don't really know. They will never know how much *one* we are in everything. They can't know what it's like. It will always be Dev and Gayle for ever—forever after—through all eternity."

There were other things he said that told me he had great insight to spiritual growth.

"I understand now a lot of things I didn't understand

before, things I can never really explain to anyone. Nor would I want to try; they are too sacred."

"Then you haven't been hurt so much that you doubt?"

"No. I've always wanted to serve Heavenly Father all my life. That's what Gayle wants, too. If this is one of the sacrifices, we can stand this."

"He watches over us in ways we can't foresee. Do you know your father checked into your insurance again, this time for Gayle? Quite miraculously, while you were on your mission your boss changed the coverage. Your health insurance used to cover about seventy percent of the costs, and with what your bills will be, you could really have been wiped out. The new policy gives full coverage for Gayle's specific case."

"That's a relief. I don't know what the bills will be, but they must be close to a hundred and fifty thousand dollars with both hospitals and her specialists."

"You know, Dev, I feel very humbled at the detailed organization of our Heavenly Father. We really have been blessed. But now we had better get some sleep or we will never get through tomorrow."

I kissed him and knew it was time to go to bed before I started crying. I felt that I had earned a good cry, and I was going to have it, but not now. There was still a lot to be done and Dev still needed help, not tears.

16

On the morning of the funeral we arrived at the chapel an hour ahead of schedule, but there were people waiting there to meet us. Dev was already greeting them when I pinned a flower on his lapel. The room was filled with relatives, and the line of friends began to form down the hall, through the corridor, and down another hall. Their presence gave me a sustaining power of love, and I gained strength from each warm embrace, each handshake, and every tear that fell. I didn't know how Dev was feeling, but I could see he was so busy comforting those who came to express sympathy that he didn't have time to think about himself. I was grateful for that.

As the time arrived for the family prayer, the announcement was made that only family members were invited to stay. Then I heard the request again, and realized that those in charge didn't know what a big group of close relatives we had. Milt hurried to inform them.

After the family prayer we joined the throngs in the chapel, where beautiful piano music was being played. Dev had asked a friend of his to play the piano instead of the organ because Gayle had always loved piano music the best. The medley of hymns filled the building like a symphony of tender exaltation. As we all took our places, the music came to an end and there was silence, an almost unbelievable silence for such a very large group of people. Then the bishop began the meeting.

As our dear, tenderhearted bishop struggled with his emotions, he said one thing that really stood out in my mind: ''The tears that I shed aren't for Gayle; I guess they are more from the knowledge I have that things are right and proper in the eyes of God even though we may not understand everything that we need to know and are going to learn eventually about our own lives here on earth." Lack of understanding—that is the cause of all our tests. We have so much to learn!

Judy's husband, Neal, gave the opening prayer. His voice was clear and controlled, and his words were soothing and full of love. "We are grateful, Father," he said, "for this beautiful daughter of thine and for the blessing it has been in our lives to know her. For during the short years she has been on this earth we have gained much. She has taught us much and we pray that each of us may remember her example, her life, and the things that she stood for, so that our lives may be enriched because of hers." I thought of the beautiful example Gayle had set in her actions, even in her suffering, and knew that many lives had already been enriched because of her.

As others rose to speak and to sing, I was filled by the air of courage, brightness, and hope that prevailed. Reviewing the events of Gayle's life was not heartbreaking. Rather, it was uplifting, inspiring, as we knew that each special thing she had done would draw her that much closer to her Father in heaven. I felt more gratitude than grief.

Gayle's Beehive girls sang the song she had taught them. Dev had asked that they remain standing after the song so he could present each of them with a gift. The gifts were the favors Gayle had prepared for them on that last day, when her lesson had been interrupted as she left for the hospital. As he presented each girl with her remembrance, he kissed each one on the cheek. He knew how Gayle had worried and prayed and loved those girls, and he wanted them to have the favor she had made to help them remember her teachings.

Then it was Dev's turn to take the stand. I had wondered if it would be wise for him to participate, but he had insisted. "It's got to be said," he had told me, "and I'm the one to say it."

There was a little tremble in Dev's voice as he thanked everyone for the love they had shown to Gayle and the way they had touched his life. Then he unfolded a paper and began to read:

"A Letter to My Eternal Bride:
"My sweetheart, as I sit here pondering all that has happened, I reflect back on you, your personality and the many blessings we've had together. It is impossible for anyone to know the happiness that we shared. My arms are empty but my heart is full with the many things you have given me. Your strength has made me strong so I feel that I can endure anything. I have gained confidence in myself by being at your side. My Gayle, I thank you for your understanding, leadership, and patience. You have always understood when I needed a special heart to cry out to. I thank you, Gayle, for waiting on your parents' couch when I would come home early in the morning from a job. It couldn't have been too comfortable sleeping there in your clothes, and yet you always asked me how the job went with no thought of what you had experienced while I was away. I thank you for waiting for me at home late at night when I would come home and find the house spotless, the table set with candlelight, and you with arms open wide to greet me. Not just a few times, but every time I came home late. My darling, how can I express to you my feelings when I was with you and the love I felt when you would get up extra early in the morning and get your cleaning done so you could go with me in the truck all day. You inspired me, reading from the *Ensign* between drives. Gayle, thanks to you, our house, no matter where it was, was sanctified. Your spirit and good attitude made our home a place of peace and refuge. Oh, Gayle, how I want to express to you my feelings for giving to me the most precious thing I could ever want, next to your love: a baby son. Now, my sweetheart, you have accepted a call from your Father in heaven to serve him. I know you will work hard and I know we will be together in spirit just as we were when I was on my mission. The preparation for

your mission was hard, but now your rewards shall be great. My helper, my karate partner, my traveling companion, my truck driver, my chef, my secretary, my comfort, my friend, my love, the mother of my children, my eternal bride, I give to you now all the love within me. Take care of Skyler.

"Forever, Your Devro."

I knew Gayle was proud of Dev at that moment. He had shown that he had the strength to endure until they could be together again—forever. Their friends Chris and Becky Harding stood up next to sing a song they had written especially for this occasion, and I could almost hear Dev and Gayle echoing the beautiful words:

Forever After

He: Once we walked hand in hand,
         Sharing our dreams and plans;
         We were together, it seemed like forever,
         But now you're so far away.

She: But we'll do the best we can—
         Someday you'll understand—
         And we'll be together forever and ever;
         It's not so far away.

Chorus

He: It's going to be so hard without you,
She: But I know you'll make it through,
He: It's going to be so hard without you,
She: But I'll be waiting for you;
Both: Then I'm going to live the best I can
         So I can be there with you
         Oh, I'll be so happy when I can see you again.

He: Then we'll walk hand in hand,
         Sharing our dreams and plans,
         We'll be together forever and ever—
         But it seems so far away.

She: But we'll be so happy here,

No more troubles and fears,
Sharing together forever and ever,
It's not so far away.
                    Chorus

The words of the song continued singing in my heart as I listened to the closing prayer. Music from the piano accompanied us again as we moved out of the chapel into the sunlight, and the sound was as near like what the angels might play as anything I'd ever heard. I thought of the words of our friend: "We asked for blessings for Gayle, even a miracle, but the real miracle is that Dev is able to survive this whole experience."

Outside the chapel I watched Devro climb into the front of the car that was carrying the casket. The funeral director had thought it strange that Dev would want to ride with the casket, but he had wanted to stay with Gayle until the last moment. There was no droop in his shoulders as he climbed into the car—no evidence of grief on his face. He was sustained and strong now, while he felt Gayle's spirit close, but there would undoubtedly be more tests ahead, times when he wouldn't feel her sustaining influence as he did now. There would be days of darkness, as there had been in the hospital, days of hurting and days of loneliness so acute that I wondered how he would stand it. But he would. He would be able to stand it because he would lean on his faith in his Father in heaven in the future as he had done in the past, and he would complete his mission on earth just as Gayle and Skyler had completed theirs, no matter how long or short the time. They were a family now, Gayle and Skyler on the other side of the veil and Devro here. Together they would accomplish their eternal goals as a family, a family that had its beginning that day in the temple when they were married and sealed for time and all eternity.

As for me—I was at peace. All our prayers for Gayle, Devro, and Skyler had been answered. They had been answered in a way that we couldn't completely understand in this existence, but I knew with a sureness that went beyond belief that when the veil was lifted, when we could see from the other side, we would be eternally grateful for this experience.

And in that magic moment of flashing wisdom, in the light of the summer sun, I felt a new understanding of the love our Heavenly Father has for us: a love so great, so beyond our mortal comprehension, that I felt I could almost hear him say:

"I'm here, my children. I'm listening and taking care of all your needs in the best way for you. Please trust me. Endure this hurt, and remember that these small hurts are nothing in comparison to the blessings I will pour out upon you if you will only trust me. For just this little while, trust me, and learn and grow from each difficult experience. I'm here—believe me—and I love you so much. Let me bless you beyond your understanding just for now . . ."

Yes, this time would pass, our deep wounds would sometime cease to bleed, and in time, when healing began to take place within his aching heart, there would be someone else for Devro. Someone would love him and give him more children, and the love he would have for her would be even stronger because of his love for Gayle because wisdom gained from endurance increases our capacity for love. But for now he would have to remember and withstand this loss. And he could, because Devro and Gayle had no regrets to mar the beauty of their union, no harsh words or unkindness to try to forget. They had only deep respect for each other—a respect that begets deep emotion. Their love had been born, lived, and tested, and would endure forever after.